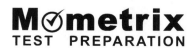

FREE Study Skills Videos/DVD Offer

Dear Customer,

Thank you for your purchase from Mometrix! We consider it an honor and a privilege that you have purchased our product and we want to ensure your satisfaction.

As part of our ongoing effort to meet the needs of test takers, we have developed a set of Study Skills Videos that we would like to give you for <u>FREE</u>. These videos cover our *best practices* for getting ready for your exam, from how to use our study materials to how to best prepare for the day of the test.

All that we ask is that you email us with feedback that would describe your experience so far with our product. Good, bad, or indifferent, we want to know what you think!

To get your FREE Study Skills Videos, you can use the **QR code** below, or send us an **email** at <u>studyvideos@mometrix.com</u> with *FREE VIDEOS* in the subject line and the following information in the body of the email:

- The name of the product you purchased.
- Your product rating on a scale of 1-5, with 5 being the highest rating.
- Your feedback. It can be long, short, or anything in between. We just want to know your impressions and experience so far with our product. (Good feedback might include how our study material met your needs and ways we might be able to make it even better. You could highlight features that you found helpful or features that you think we should add.)

If you have any questions or concerns, please don't hesitate to contact me directly.

Thanks again!

Sincerely,

Jay Willis
Vice President
jay.willis@mometrix.com
1-800-673-8175

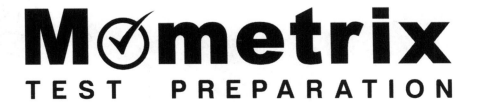

Psychiatric-Mental Health Nurse Practitioner Exam Practice Questions

NP Practice Tests & Exam Review for the Nurse Practitioner Exam

Written and edited by the Mometrix Test Prep

Printed in the United States of America

This paper meets the requirements of ANSI/NISO Z39.48-1992 (Permanence of Paper).

Mometrix offers volume discount pricing to institutions. For more information or a price quote, please contact our sales department at sales@mometrix.com or 888-248-1219.

Mometrix Media LLC is not affiliated with or endorsed by any official testing organization. All organizational and test names are trademarks of their respective owners.

Paperback
ISBN 13: 978-1-5167-0751-5
ISBN 10: 1-5167-0751-6

Ebook
ISBN 13: 978-1-5167-0939-7
ISBN 10: 1-5167-0939-X

DEAR FUTURE EXAM SUCCESS STORY

First of all, **THANK YOU** for purchasing Mometrix study materials!

Second, congratulations! You are one of the few determined test-takers who are committed to doing whatever it takes to excel on your exam. **You have come to the right place.** We developed these practice tests with one goal in mind: to deliver you the best possible approximation of the questions you will see on test day.

Standardized testing is one of the biggest obstacles on your road to success, which only increases the importance of doing well in the high-pressure, high-stakes environment of test day. Your results on this test could have a significant impact on your future, and these practice tests will give you the repetitions you need to build your familiarity and confidence with the test content and format to help you achieve your full potential on test day.

Your success is our success

We would love to hear from you! If you would like to share the story of your exam success or if you have any questions or comments in regard to our products, please contact us at **800-673-8175** or **support@mometrix.com**.

Thanks again for your business and we wish you continued success!

Sincerely,
The Mometrix Test Preparation Team

TABLE OF CONTENTS

Practice Test #1

1. The concepts of defense mechanisms, transference and counter transference that are used in psychiatric mental health nursing practice are derived from which of the following theories?

    a. Psychosocial theory
    b. Humanistic theory
    c. Psychodynamic theory
    d. Cognitive theory

2. Which of the following stages is not a component of the transtheoretical model of behavior change?

    a. Pre-contemplation
    b. Contemplation
    c. Action
    d. Acceptance

3. A PMHNP is seeing a client that is working to change a problematic behavior. At his last visit, the client states that on a daily basis, he is working to prevent the problematic behavior as he has seen positive changes that have occurred in his life as a result of changing the behavior. Based on the transtheoretical model of behavior change, which of the following stages is this client in?

    a. Preparation
    b. Maintenance
    c. Termination
    d. Contemplation

4. Which of the following nursing theorists is considered to be the founder of psychiatric nursing?

    a. Dorothea Orem
    b. Betty Neuman
    c. Martha Rogers
    d. Hildegard Peplau

5. The unit manager of an inpatient psychiatric unit asks the mental health nurse practitioner to conduct an in-service with the new registered nurses on the unit to teach the about evidence-based practice. The NP decides to utilize the commonly used PICO model as a guide to assist the new staff. What does the "C" in the PICO model stand for?

    a. Comparison
    b. Clinician
    c. Compliance
    d. Clarification

6. A psychiatric nurse practitioner in a large academic medication center has noticed recently that there has been an increase in violent behaviors of patients with psychiatric illnesses hospitalized outside of the psychiatric unit. The NP would like to review the literature on behavioral response teams and their effectiveness in assisting non-behavioral health staff in managing this type of behavior. Now that the NP has begun the inquiry process, what is the next step in the evidence-based practice process?

    a. Search for the best evidence.
    b. Evaluate outcomes.
    c. Ask clinical questions using patient scenarios.
    d. Integrate the clinical evidence into practice.

7. Which of the following is not a key component of evidence-based practice?

    a. Clinical expertise
    b. Personal experience
    c. Research evidence
    d. Patient values

8. The ability to transform a disastrous situation into a growth experience in an effort to move forward is defined as which of the following?

    a. Concordance
    b. Adaptation
    c. Resilience
    d. Self-efficacy

9. Which of the following concepts is defined as the process of developing a mutually agreed upon treatment plan?

    a. Adherence
    b. Concordance
    c. Compliance
    d. Patient-centered care

10. Which of the following best describes "culturally competent" care?

    a. The clinical skills/professional behaviors of a clinician that focus on the cultural beliefs, values, and perceptions of the patient during the therapeutic relationship established between the patient and clinician.
    b. A way of life belonging to an individual or group of individuals that reflects values and customs.
    c. Recognition that each individual is unique along the dimensions of race, gender, ethnicity, religious beliefs, and sexual orientation.
    d. The adoption of the elements of one culture by members of a different culture.

11. Which of the following is not an example of a monoamine neurotransmitter?

    a. Dopamine
    b. Serotonin
    c. Norepinephrine
    d. Acetylcholine

12. Which of the following neurotransmitters is implicated in the regulation of sleep, mood, pain, and appetite?

    a. Glutamate
    b. Norepinephrine
    c. Serotonin
    d. Gamma-aminobutyric acid

13. Which of the following is a molecule with the same effect on the postsynaptic neuron as the neurotransmitter itself?

    a. Antagonist
    b. Agonist
    c. Receptor
    d. Synapse

14. Which two neurotransmitters can be grouped together into the catecholamine category due to sharing a commonality in having the same core biochemical structure (the catechol group)?

    a. Norepinephrine and histamine
    b. Dopamine and norepinephrine
    c. Serotonin and epinephrine
    d. Dopamine and serotonin

15. Which of the following antipsychotics is classified as moderate potency?

    a. Thioridazine
    b. Chlorpromazine
    c. Haloperidol
    d. Loxapine

16. A mental health nurse practitioner is working in an inpatient psychiatric unit and is called to see a newly admitted patient. The patient is a 32-year-old schizophrenic currently being treated with haloperidol. The patient was brought to the Emergency Department by her mother who states that earlier in the day the patient became very confused and agitated. The registered nurse caring for the patient states that the patient is diaphoretic with a heart rate running in the 140's and a temperature of 39.0 °C. The patient's lab work shows an elevated white blood count and an elevation in creatine phosphokinase. Which of the following conditions might the patient be experiencing?

    a. Extrapyramidal side effects
    b. Cardiometabolic syndrome
    c. Neuroleptic malignant syndrome
    d. Serotonin syndrome

17. Which of the following pharmacologic options may be considered in the treatment of neuroleptic malignant syndrome in patients that do not respond to the discontinuation of the neuroleptic agent and supportive care within the first day or two?

    a. Benztropine
    b. Atropine
    c. Chlorpromazine
    d. Dantrolene

18. Which of the following conditions shares many of the common features of neuroleptic malignant syndrome (NMS) and may be difficult to clinically distinguish from NMS?

    a. Malignant catatonia
    b. Cardiometabolic syndrome
    c. Tardive dyskinesia
    d. Akathisia

19. Which of the following is not a common physical finding in patients with suspected selective serotonin syndrome?

    a. Hyperthermia
    b. Agitation
    c. Decreased bowel sounds
    d. Akathisia

20. Which of the following medications may be administered as an antidote in patients with selective serotonin syndrome?

    a. Bromocriptine
    b. Propranolol
    c. Cyproheptadine
    d. Dantrolene

21. According to the DSM-5-TR, catatonia is a behavioral syndrome that occurs in ill individuals with an underlying psychiatric or general medical disorder. It is characterized by the predominant presence of at least three of the clinical criteria defined in the DSM-5-TR Which of the following is not part of the clinical criteria used to define catatonia?

    a. Akathisia
    b. Negativism
    c. Echolalia
    d. Posturing

22. Which of the following laboratory findings does not correlate with a diagnosis of malignant catatonia?

    a. White blood cell count of 15,000
    b. Serum bicarbonate level of 18 mmol/L
    c. Creatinine kinase of 1200 IU/L
    d. Serum iron level of 30 mcg/dL

23. A mental health nurse practitioner is rounding on a patient on the inpatient psychiatry unit that was admitted with a diagnosis of bipolar disorder. In speaking with the patient's registered nurse, she shares with the NP that on admission the patient is verbally unresponsive and has been staring at the wall across from his bed, lying in the same position since he arrived. In addition, the patient is resistant to any type of movement and is not following any type of instructions. Which of the following sub-types of catatonia is consistent with the patient's clinical presentation?

    a. Excited catatonia
    b. Neuroleptic malignant syndrome
    c. Retarded catatonia
    d. Malignant catatonia

24. Which of the following pharmacologic therapies is recommended for patients with bipolar disorder that present with acute hypomania or mild to moderate manic symptoms?

   a. Risperidone or olanzapine monotherapy
   b. Lithium and Ziprasidone
   c. Lithium and Valproate
   d. Lamotrigine monotherapy

25. The FDA recommends screening for the HLA-B*1502 allele in patients of Asian descent, prior to the initiation of which pharmacologic agent used in the treatment of bipolar disorder?

   a. Valproate
   b. Lithium
   c. Risperidone
   d. Carbamazepine

26. A mental health NP is rounding on a patient that is scheduled to undergo electroconvulsive therapy (ECT). Which of the following statements by the patient indicates a need for further instruction/education?

   a. "ECT causes chemical changes in my brain that may help my depression."
   b. "I should continue taking my Ativan prior to my ECT treatment."
   c. "I know that I may feel confused after I wake up from my ECT treatment."
   d. "I should take my blood pressure medication with a sip of water 2 hours prior to my ECT treatment."

27. Which of the following clinical findings would NOT be expected to be seen in a patient that is experiencing lithium toxicity?

   a. Nausea and vomiting
   b. Confusion
   c. Prolonged QTc interval
   d. Elevation in cardiac biomarkers

28. Which of the following is the recommended therapeutic concentration of lithium?

   a. 1.0-1.5 mEq/L
   b. 0.8-1.2 mEq/L
   c. 0.2-.06 mEq/L
   d. 1.5-2.0 mEq/L

29. The PMHNP is completing a physical assessment on an outpatient with bipolar disorder who is currently taking lithium. The NP reviews the patient's lab work and note a sub-therapeutic lithium level. Which of the following statements made by the patient may have had an impact on decreasing the patient's lithium level?

   a. "I have been ill over the past few days with a high fever."
   b. "I have been advised by my cardiologist to decrease my sodium intake so I have reduced my daily sodium intake."
   c. "My primary care physician is concerned that my kidneys are not functioning properly."
   d. "I know I need to watch my salt intake. I have recently been eating foods with a higher amount of sodium."

30. Which of the following medications interacts with lithium and may cause a decrease in the serum lithium level?

    a. Ibuprofen
    b. Metronidazole
    c. Lisinopril
    d. Theophylline

31. Psychotherapy uses similar pathways to pharmacotherapy, but works in a top-down manner as opposed to a bottom down manner. The pathway psychotherapy uses is:

    a. Limbic system, prefrontal cortex
    b. Hippocampus, amygdala
    c. Prefrontal cortex, limbic system
    d. Thalamus, prefrontal cortex

32. Which of the following complementary therapies increases serotonin levels, alters dopamine function, and regulates corticotrophin-releasing factor?

    a. Valerian
    b. Folate
    c. Omega-3 fatty acids
    d. Ginseng

33. Which of the following supplements/alternate therapies may be utilized to enhance sleep?

    a. Gingko biloba
    b. Ginseng
    c. St. John's wort
    d. Valerian

34. Which of the following statements is not true regarding transcranial magnetic stimulation?

    a. Treatment typically involves daily administration for 4-6 weeks.
    b. The procedure does not require any medication or anesthesia.
    c. Cognitive side effects of transcranial magnetic stimulation are similar to those experienced in ECT treatment.
    d. Treatment is expensive and insurance reimbursement may be difficult to obtain.

35. Vagal nerve stimulation is an uncommonly used treatment option for patients with severely and chronically treatment resistant depressive disorders. Which of the following disorders is vagal nerve stimulation also utilized for the treatment of?

    a. Attention deficit/hyperactivity disorder
    b. Insomnia
    c. Medically refractory partial onset seizures
    d. Migraine headaches

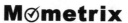

36. Which of the following cranial nerves is associated with the "facial" anticholinergic effects of dry mouth, decreased respiratory secretions and decreased tearing?

    a. VII
    b. III
    c. IX
    d. X

37. Which of the following medications is approved by the United States FDA for the treatment of bulimia nervosa?

    a. Brofaromine
    b. Isocarboxazid
    c. Sertraline
    d. Fluoxetine

38. A mental health nurse practitioner is rounding on a 17-year-old patient admitted to the inpatient unit with a diagnosis of anorexia nervosa. The patient has recently experienced a significant weight loss and her current treatment plan includes a re-feeding plan with a goal of gaining 1-2 pounds per week. The NP is providing education to the patient and her family about re-feeding syndrome. Which of the following is NOT a characteristic of re-feeding syndrome?

    a. Fluid overload
    b. Hyperkalemia
    c. Glucose intolerance
    d. Thiamine deficiency

39. Which of the following has the highest death rate of all the psychiatric disorders?

    a. Bulimia nervosa
    b. Major depression
    c. Anorexia nervosa
    d. Schizophrenia

40. All of the following clinical features are more commonly seen in patients with bipolar major depression as opposed to unipolar major depression EXCEPT for:

    a. Hypersomnia
    b. Leaden paralysis
    c. Hallucinations
    d. Greater ability to function socially

41. Which of the following statements regarding bipolar disorder in a geriatric patient is NOT true?

    a. Comorbid general medical disorders are more common in the older adult.
    b. Excessive sexual interest/behavior is less common in older adults during manic/hypomanic episodes.
    c. Comorbid anxiety disorders and substance use disorders are more common in the geriatric population.
    d. Cognitive impairment is more common and severe in the geriatric population.

42. A PMHNP is seeing a patient in the outpatient clinic with a diagnosis of bipolar I disorder. During the patient interview he states that over the past four days he has not slept much and has not really felt tired. The NP notices that the patient is more talkative than usual and is not allowing any periods of silence during the interview process. He appears irritable and easily distracted. The patient mentions that he and his wife have been arguing frequently, most recently due to a couple of shopping trips that he made where he spent several hundred dollars. The patient makes the comment that he has always felt that "he could have done better" and his wife is not worthy of being married to him anyways. The patient states that he has been going to work as normal and has been exceptionally productive over the past couple of days. Which of the following diagnoses is the patient likely experiencing?

   a. Manic episode
   b. Bipolar major depression
   c. Hypomanic episode
   d. Mood episode with mixed features

43. All of the following classifications of medications have the potential to induce psychosis EXCEPT:

   a. Corticosteroids
   b. Antivirals
   c. Anticholinergics
   d. Anticoagulants

44. A mental health nurse practitioner is working on an inpatient psychiatry unit and one of the new registered nurses tells her that she is caring for a patient with a diagnosis of a manic episode with mixed features. She asks the NP to explain what this means. The NP advises the nurse that patients experiencing episodes of bipolar mania, hypomania and major depression can also experience symptoms of the opposite polarity (mixed features) and that a manic episode with mixed features is defined as an episode that meets the diagnostic criteria for mania along with at least three of the defined symptoms being present on most days of the episode. Which of the following is NOT included in the defined symptoms associated with a manic episode with mixed features?

   a. Depressed mood
   b. Low energy
   c. Flight of ideas
   d. Recurrent thoughts about death or suicide or a suicide attempt

45. Which of the following statements is true regarding mood episodes with mixed features?

   a. Response to treatment is often greater in mood episodes with mixed features as opposed to pure mania or pure bipolar major depression.
   b. Patients with mixed features are at greater risk for suicidal ideation and behavior.
   c. Mixed features occur infrequently.
   d. It is common for mood episodes with mixed features to transition to mania.

46. Which of the following defense mechanisms is associated with a lower level of adaptation and maturity?

   a. Altruism
   b. Somatization
   c. Sublimation
   d. Humor

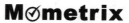

47. The defense mechanism of reacting to unacceptable impulses or thoughts as if outside of oneself is known as:

   a. Distortion
   b. Intellectualization
   c. Dissociation
   d. Projection

48. Failure to thrive (FTT) is believed to be one manifestation of depression in infancy. Which of the following is NOT a characteristic of failure to thrive?

   a. Psychomotor delay
   b. Weight below the 10th percentile on body charts
   c. Iron deficiency
   d. Feeding problems with no identified disease process

49. Which of the following treatment options might be appropriate for a patient diagnosed with severe depression without psychotic symptoms?

   a. Selective serotonin reuptake inhibitor
   b. Psychotherapy
   c. Inpatient hospitalization
   d. All of the above

50. Which of the following treatment options would NOT be appropriate for a patient with severe depression and a history of polarity?

   a. Omega-3 fatty acid
   b. Mood stabilizer
   c. Self-help
   d. Social rhythm therapy

51. Which of the following symptoms would NOT be classified as a positive symptom in patients with schizophrenia?

   a. Patient reports hearing voices.
   b. Patient reports seeing human faces.
   c. Patient reports being visited by aliens.
   d. Patient reports a lack of energy.

52. Which of the following statements is NOT true regarding deficit schizophrenia?

   a. Patients are less likely to experience delusions with high emotional content.
   b. Patients are more likely to have a depressive disorder.
   c. Patients are less likely to show improvement.
   d. Patients are less likely to have a substance use disorder.

53. Which of the following neurological "soft signs" is defined as the inability to recognize familiar objects by touch alone?

   a. Akathisia
   b. Astereognosis
   c. Right-left confusion
   d. Agraphesthesia

54. Which of the following metabolic disturbances is associated with schizophrenia?

    a. Hypertension
    b. Hyperlipidemia
    c. Diabetes
    d. All of the above

55. Which of the following disorders is diagnosed when all of the DSM-5-TR criteria for schizophrenia are met but the total duration of the disorder is less than six months?

    a. Schizoaffective disorder
    b. Bipolar disorder
    c. Schizophreniform disorder
    d. Major depression with psychotic features

56. A mental health nurse practitioner is seeing a patient diagnosed with schizophrenia in the outpatient clinic. The patient experienced an inadequate response to his prescribed antipsychotic medication. The patient's medication was trialed for a period of eight weeks, reaching the maximum tolerated dose (within the therapeutic range). The NP is concerned that the patient may be "treatment resistant." Which of the following interventions is not an appropriate next step in this patient's treatment plan?

    a. Start the patient on a clozapine trial.
    b. Optimize the current antipsychotic drug treatment.
    c. Assess the patient for other causes of residual schizophrenia symptoms.
    d. Optimize non-pharmacologic interventions.

57. Prior to the initiation of clozapine, the patient's absolute neutrophil count should be greater than or equal to:

    a. 2000 cells/microliter
    b. 500 cells/microliter
    c. 1500 cells/microliter
    d. 1000 cells/microliter

58. Which of the following statements is NOT true regarding neutrophil monitoring in patients taking clozapine?

    a. Neutrophil monitoring should be conducted weekly during the first six months of clozapine administration.
    b. Neutrophil monitoring should be conducted every other week for the second six months of clozapine administration.
    c. After one year of therapy, neutrophil monitoring should be conducted every four weeks for the duration of the therapy.
    d. Neutrophil monitoring should be conducted every 3 weeks for the duration of the therapy.

59. A patient diagnosed with treatment-resistant schizophrenia was started on clozapine 4 weeks ago. During today's office visit, the patient's absolute neutrophil count (ANC) comes back at 1200 cells/mcL. Which of the following is the most appropriate next step in this patient's treatment plan?

    a. Continue the clozapine and weekly absolute neutrophil count checks.
    b. Continue the clozapine and increase the absolute neutrophil count checks to three times per week.
    c. Hold clozapine treatment until the absolute neutrophil count rises to 1500.
    d. Discontinue the clozapine.

60. All of the following laboratory tests should be monitored weekly in patients receiving clozapine for the first four weeks of therapy EXCEPT for:

    a. Eosinophil count
    b. C-reactive protein
    c. Fasting blood glucose
    d. Troponin

61. Which of the following clinical presentations is not usually associated with a primary psychiatric (psychotic) disorder?

    a. Auditory hallucinations
    b. Family history often present
    c. Onset in forties or older
    d. Insidious onset

62. Which of the following subtypes of delusional disorders is the most common?

    a. Grandiose
    b. Mixed
    c. Persecutory
    d. Erotomanic

63. Which of the following is the most common form of monosymptomatic hypochondriacal psychosis?

    a. Delusions of dysmorphism
    b. Delusions of parasitosis
    c. Delusions of halitosis
    d. Delusions of body odor

64. A mental health nurse practitioner is preparing to prescribe a serotonin norepinephrine reuptake inhibitor (SNRI) for a patient with a history of hypertension. Which SNRI would be the most appropriate choice given the patient's history?

    a. Duloxetine
    b. Venlafaxine
    c. Desvenlafaxine
    d. Milnacipran

65. A PMHNP has just finished providing education to a patient that has been prescribed a serotonin norepinephrine reuptake inhibitor (SNRI) for. Which of the following statements by the patient indicates a need for further clarification?

    a. "I know that I cannot abruptly stop taking this medication."
    b. "I know that this medication may cause sexual dysfunction."
    c. "I know that a full response may take many weeks"
    d. "I know that I should take my SNRI on an empty stomach."

66. The enzyme monoamine oxidase has two forms, MAO-A and MAO-B. MAO-A is responsible for:

    a. The breakdown of serotonin and norepinephrine
    b. Metabolization of phenylethylamine
    c. Breakdown of dopamine
    d. Blockade of monoamine oxidase

67. Which of the following food items should be strictly prohibited in patients taking monoamine oxidase inhibitors?

    a. Sour cream
    b. Gorgonzola cheese
    c. Red wine
    d. Caffeine-containing drinks

68. Which of the following is NOT true regarding the use of the selegiline patch for the treatment of depression?

    a. Dose increases should occur in increments of 3 mg/day at a minimum interval of at least 2 weeks.
    b. The maximum dose of the selegiline transdermal patch is 15 mg/day.
    c. There are no diet restrictions when the selegiline patch is used at the 6 mg/day dosage.
    d. The transdermal delivery of selegiline allows for avoidance of direct inhibition of MAO-A in the gastrointestinal tract.

69. A mental health nurse practitioner is seeing a 22-year-old female patient in the outpatient clinic who presents today reporting that she is experiencing mild to moderate anxiety over the fear of an undiagnosed brain tumor. The patient's mother reports that the patient has been preoccupied with thoughts that she has a brain tumor for the past seven months. The patient reports that the only physical symptom that she is experiencing is an occasional mild headache. The patient's mother reports that when the headaches occur the patient's anxiety is markedly increased. In addition, the patient is avoiding exercising due to the fear that it will cause the brain tumor to bleed. The patient's mother states that radiologic findings have confirmed that the patient does not have evidence of any type of brain lesion or tumor. Which of the following DSM-5-TR diagnoses might this patient meet the criteria for?

    a. Functional neurological symptom disorder
    b. Illness anxiety disorder
    c. Hypochondriasis
    d. Somatoform disorder

70. Pharmacotherapy may be utilized as a third line treatment option for patients with conversion disorder. Which of the following agents are most commonly used for the treatment of conversion disorder?

    a. Anticonvulsants
    b. Benzodiazepines
    c. Antidepressants
    d. Hydroxyzine

71. Which of the following medications is indicated for a patient with alcohol intoxication that has become agitated and violent?

    a. Droperidol
    b. Lorazepam
    c. Risperidone
    d. Midazolam

72. The mnemonic "FIND ME" can be utilized to help a clinician determine the etiology of acute delirium and violence. What does the "M" in "FIND ME" stand for?

    a. Mania
    b. Methamphetamine
    c. Metabolic
    d. Mental state

73. A mental health nurse practitioner is working in a busy emergency room. A 20-year-old male patient arrives to the emergency department via ambulance. His roommate accompanied the patient to the hospital. The patient is extremely agitated and violent, yelling out and trying to hit the staff. The patient's roommate states that the patient took "a bunch of spice gold" a few hours ago and started shortly after to hallucinate and become agitated. Physical assessment reveals a temperature of 102 °F, BP 88/40, HR 140, and RR 24. Lab results show a serum potassium level of 6.2 and a serum creatinine kinase of 10500 U/L. Based on the patient's clinical presentation which of the following clinical conditions might the patient be experiencing?

    a. Dystonia
    b. Sepsis
    c. Neuroleptic malignant syndrome
    d. Rhabdomyolysis

74. A mental health nurse practitioner in an emergency room receives a 27-year-old female patient who presents to the E.D. with complaints of chest pain and diaphoresis. Physical assessment reveals a blood pressure of 190/100, HR 148, RR 26, and the patient seems mildly agitated. When returning to see the patient a few minutes later the nurse practitioner find that she has become much more agitated and is experiencing hallucinations. The patient's boyfriend states "She probably took some more of that lunar wave stuff. This is how she gets when she takes that stuff." The NP is suspecting that the patient is suffering from a synthetic cathinone overdose. Which of the following interventions might be considered in the treatment of a cathinone overdose?

    a. Gastric lavage
    b. Administration of 2 mg of IV lorazepam
    c. Begin a nitroprusside drip at 10mcg/kg/minute
    d. Administration of 5 mg of IV haloperidol

75. A mental health nurse practitioner receives a 45-year-old female patient who presents to the E.D. with agitation, confusion, and blurred vision. Upon physical examination the NP notes that the patient's skin is very warm and dry and she has extreme facial flushing. Pupils are dilated, and the patient is tachycardiac with a heart rate of 150. Temperature is 101.5 °F. Bowels sounds are absent and the patient has marked distension over the urinary bladder. Which of the following conditions is suspected?

    a. Serotonin toxicity
    b. Salicylate poisoning
    c. Anticholinergic poisoning
    d. Sympathomimetic overdose

76. Which of the following atypical antidepressants is the least likely to interact with other medications?

    a. Bupropion
    b. Mirtazapine
    c. Agomelatine
    d. Maprotiline

77. Which of the following diagnoses is contraindicated in the use of bupropion?

    a. Pregnancy
    b. Active liver disease
    c. Bulimia nervosa
    d. Heart failure

78. Which of the following statements is true regarding transient global amnesia (TGA)?

    a. A past history of a similar episode is common.
    b. The mean duration of episodes is approximately 2 hours.
    c. Triggering events are common and may include acute emotional events and physical events as well as chronic emotional stress.
    d. TGA attacks rarely have a well-defined time of onset.

79. Current theories surrounding the pathophysiology of transient global amnesia include all of the following EXCEPT:

    a. Migraines
    b. Psychogenic disorder
    c. Venous congestion
    d. Arterial insufficiency

80. Which of the following second-generation antipsychotics carries the least risk of cardiac arrhythmias?

    a. Ziprasidone
    b. Olanzapine
    c. Aripiprazole
    d. Quetiapine

81. Which of the following agents has NOT shown promise as a neuroprotective agent in the treatment of Parkinson's disease?

    a. Vitamin E
    b. Selegiline
    c. Rasagiline
    d. Coenzyme Q10

82. Which of the following is NOT one of the six principles of trauma informed care according to Substance Abuse and Mental Health Services Administration (SAMHSA)?

    a. Safety
    b. Trustworthiness and transparency
    c. Communication
    d. Peer support

83. Which of the following statements is not true regarding the DSM-5-TR diagnosis of psychological factors affecting other medical conditions (PFAOMC)?

    a. Psychological or behavioral factors do not pose any additional health risks to the patient.
    b. Other mental disorders do not explain the psychological or behavioral factors.
    c. A general medical symptom or disorder is present.
    d. Psychological or behavioral factors disrupt the treatment of the general medical condition.

84. A patient being seen in the outpatient clinic was recently diagnosed with psoriatic arthritis. The patient is now experiencing a significant amount of anxiety related to her diagnosis. She has become increasingly more isolated and is spending less time with her friends. Which of the following diagnoses might be considered?

    a. Psychological factors affecting other medical conditions (PFAOMC)
    b. Illness anxiety disorder
    c. Conversion disorder
    d. Adjustment disorder

85. Under the Health Insurance Portability and Accountability Act (HIPAA), adolescents are considered "individuals" (enabling them to obtain access to their medical records, obtain copies and request corrections, and authorize the disclosure of private health information) under three distinct circumstances. Which of the following circumstances is not included in this rule establishing adolescents as individuals?

    a. When the parent is the patient's representative and provides consent in conjunction with the minor patient
    b. When the minor has the right to consent to health care and does consent
    c. When the minor may legally receive care without parental consent and the minor or a third party (i.e., court) can consent to the care
    d. When a parent is in agreement with a statement of confidentiality between the healthcare provider and the minor patient and this is formally documented in the medical record

86. Which of the following regulations allows parents access to their minor's educational records as well as any health information that is contained within those records?

    a. Confidentiality of Medical Information Act (CMIA)
    b. Health Insurance Portability and Accountability Act (HIPAA)
    c. Children's Online Privacy Protection Rule (COPPA)
    d. The Family Educational Rights and Privacy Act (FERPA)

87. Which of the following statements is not true regarding payment for healthcare services by adolescent patients?

    a. Confidentiality can be breached when a bill for healthcare services for an adolescent patient is sent to a parent or guardian for payment, regardless of whether or not the service provided was performed without parental consent.

    b. Emancipated minors have financial responsibility for healthcare services with the exception of emergency treatment.

    c. To protect confidentiality of patients, some clinics opt to not bill for certain services such as pregnancy testing or sexually transmitted disease testing.

    d. Parents are not financially liable for the healthcare services provided to a minor.

88. Which of the following is an example of a "conscience clause"?

    a. A pharmacist shall not be required to fill a prescription for an emergency contraceptive drug.

    b. State law requiring that parental consent must be obtained for minor patients seeking abortion services.

    c. A clinician must report violent injuries (including all wounds inflicted by stabbing or gunshot) regardless of confidentiality.

    d. Signing of a written confidentiality agreement between the patient and healthcare provider.

89. Which of the following symptoms in acute stress disorder is classified as an "arousal" symptom?

    a. Persistent inability to experience positive emotions

    b. Problems with concentration

    c. Dissociative reactions

    d. Recurrent, involuntary, and intrusive distressing memories of the traumatic event

90. Which of the following statements best describes sexual dysfunction in patients taking selective serotonin reuptake inhibitors (SSRI)?

    a. Recommended treatment option for patients on an SSRI who are benefiting from therapy and experience severe sexual dysfunction is augmentation of the SSRI with a second drug.

    b. A phosphodiesterase-5 inhibitor is the recommended treatment option for women with decreased libido.

    c. The estimated incidence of sexual dysfunction related to selective serotonin reuptake inhibitors (SSRI) is 30%.

    d. The recommended initial approach to patients on an SSRI that experience sexual dysfunction is to wait for spontaneous remission of sexual impairment.

91. Which of the following communication strategies would be appropriate for building empathy in developing a therapeutic client-nurse relationship?

    a. Clarification

    b. Normalizing

    c. Simple reflections

    d. Giving recognition

92. Which of the following statements best represents the use of "normalizing" as a therapeutic communication technique?

    a. "What brings you in to see me today?"

    b. "Many people tell me that when they are feeling very depressed, they sleep a lot more than usual. Has this ever happened to you?"

    c. "You are concerned about being a good wife."

    d. "Tell me how your depression affects you on a daily basis."

93. Transitioning from one topic to another in the therapeutic communication process can be challenging for a clinician. Dr. Shawn Shea described these transitions as "gates." Which of the following "gates" is best described as the return to a new area of discussion by referring back to a previous statement made by the client?

    a. Implied gate

    b. Natural gate

    c. Phantom gate

    d. Referred gate

94. During a session, a client begins to talk about her son's upcoming wedding. The PMHNP asks her "What was your wedding like?" This is an example of which type of transitional gate?

    a. Natural gate

    b. Implied gate

    c. Spontaneous gate

    d. Referred gate

95. Which of the following statements is true regarding suicide risk in patients with schizophrenia?

    a. Patients with schizophrenia have a 20-fold greater risk for suicide.

    b. Suicide attempts are made by 20-50% of patients with schizophrenia.

    c. 80% of suicides occur in the first 2 years of illness.

    d. Risk factors include female gender.

96. Sleep efficiency is defined as:

    a. Sleep stage characterized by fast frequency, low voltage mixed EEG, rapid eye movements and muscle atonia

    b. Total sleep time / time in bed (x100)

    c. Wake from sleep onset during time in bed to lights on

    d. Total minutes of NREM 1,2,3 and REM stages

97. Which of the following pharmacologic treatments may be appropriate for a patient experiencing a sleep onset insomnia?

    a. Eszopiclone

    b. Modafinil

    c. Zolpidem

    d. Ramelteon

98. Which of the following is not a typical symptom associated with narcolepsy?

a. Hallucinations at onset and end of sleep
b. Cataplexy
c. Abrupt loss of muscle tone
d. Loud snoring

99. Hormone production can adversely affect sleep. Which of the following statements is true regarding hormones and their effect on sleep?

a. Melatonin levels decrease during the day in response to sunlight exposure.
b. Cortisol is associated with arousal.
c. Melatonin levels reach a nadir near the onset of sleep.
d. Cortisol levels are increased during sleep.

100. A patient that has been diagnosed with major depression. In addition, after undergoing a sleep study, that patient was diagnosed with obstructive sleep apnea (OSA). The nurse practitioner has provided the patient with some education regarding OSA. Which of the following statements by the patient indicates a need for further education?

a. "I should avoid alcohol prior to bedtime."
b. "I should maintain a healthy weight."
c. "I should let me health care providers know that I have been diagnosed with OSA."
d. "I should sleep on my back."

101. Which of the following anti-depressants also has antipsychotic effects?

a. Maprotiline
b. Nortriptyline
c. Amoxapine
d. Doxepin

102. Which of the following cyclic antidepressants is considered the "most potent?"

a. Trimipramine
b. Doxepin
c. Amoxapine
d. Protriptyline

103. Which of the following cyclic antidepressants has the highest affinity for histamine H1 receptors and is therefore generally more sedating?

a. Doxepin
b. Protriptyline
c. Desipramine
d. Amitriptyline

104. Which of the following statements is true regarding the management of benzodiazepine overdose?

a. Gastrointestinal decontamination with activated charcoal is recommended first line treatment in benzodiazepine overdose.
b. Oral benzodiazepines taken without a co-ingestant often cause significant toxicity.
c. Most cases of isolated benzodiazepine ingestion are able to be managed successfully with supportive care.
d. The use of flumazenil is recommended in the treatment of benzodiazepine overdose.

105. A mental health nurse practitioner is rounding on a patient that has been receiving intravenous diazepam as part of an alcohol withdrawal protocol. The patient presented with severe symptoms associated with ethanol withdrawal and has required a large amount of intravenous diazepam. The registered nurse states that the patient is now hypotensive and has a significantly elevated lactic acid level. The patient is also hypoglycemic and has dark colored urine. While assessing the patient, he starts to seize. Which of the following conditions might the patient be experiencing?

    a. Propylene glycol toxicity
    b. Sepsis
    c. Gamma hydroxybutyrate (GHB) intoxication
    d. Acute renal failure

106. A patient is experiencing moderate symptoms of gamma hydroxybutyrate (GHB) withdrawal without delirium including anxiety, insomnia, and tremors. Which of the following treatment options would be most appropriate?

    a. Haloperidol
    b. Metoprolol
    c. Diazepam
    d. Outpatient detoxification

107. Which of the following symptoms is commonly seen in the clinical presentation of a patient with gamma hydroxybutyrate (GHB) intoxication?

    a. Hyperthermia
    b. Tachycardia
    c. Respiratory depression
    d. Hypertension

108. Which of the following statements does NOT accurately represent the position of the American Psychiatric Nurses Association (APNA) regarding ECT treatment?

    a. APNA is willing to assist in development of standards of practice in the proper application of ECT treatment.
    b. APNA believes that ECT operated by properly trained professionals and in circumstances of medical necessity offers severely depressed patients an option that would otherwise be unavailable.
    c. ECT is a proven therapy and further clinical trials are not needed to establish its safety and efficacy.
    d. The most significant concern about ECT treatment are the physical side effects, including the risk of serious medical complications.

109. Which of the following statements regarding a psychiatric advance directive (according to the Centers for Medicare and Medicaid Services) is NOT accurate?

    a. A psychiatric advance directive should be accorded the same respect and consideration that a traditional advance directive for health care is given.
    b. Patient wishes regarding restraint and seclusion should not be included in a psychiatric advance directive.
    c. State laws regarding the use of psychiatric advance directives vary.
    d. A psychiatric advance directive may name another person who is authorized to make decisions for an individual if deemed to be legally incompetent to make his/her own decisions.

110. According to the Centers for Medicare and Medicaid Services (CMS), an incidental use or disclosure of protected health information includes all of the following components EXCEPT which of the following?

a. It is limited in nature.
b. It cannot be reasonably prevented.
c. It is a by-product of an underlying rule or disclosure that violates the HIPAA privacy rule.
d. It occurs as a result of another use or disclosure that is permitted.

111. Which of the following examples best describes incidental use or disclosure of protected health information according to the Health Insurance Portability and Accountability Act (HIPAA)?

a. An unencrypted flash drive containing patient information is stolen from an employee's vehicle.
b. A patient's lab results were discarded in the regular trash as opposed to the secured paper shredder.
c. A patient's private health information was disclosed to a third party without a business associate agreement.
d. A patient visitor overhears a registered nurse giving report on one of her patients to another registered nurse.

112. The Health Insurance Portability and Accountability Act specifies that "patients should be allowed to inspect and obtain a copy of health information about them that is held by providers." Providers may not withhold information expect in the case of limited circumstances. These circumstances include:

a. Psychotherapy notes
b. A licensed health care professional who has determined that the access requested would likely endanger the life or physical safety of the individual or other person
c. The information containing data obtained under a promise of confidentiality (from someone other than a health care provider) when inspection could reasonably reveal the source
d. All of the above

113. Hospitals are required to inform patients and/or patient representatives of the internal grievance process, including whom to contact to file a grievance. Which of the following best describes the definition of a "patient grievance?"

a. Any written complaint regarding the patient's care or billing
b. Any written complaint regarding a patient's care not including complaints related to abuse or neglect, issues related to the hospital's compliance with the CMS conditions of participation, or a Medicare beneficiary billing complaint related to rights or limitations
c. Information obtained from patient satisfaction surveys
d. A formal or informal written or verbal complaint regarding the patient's care that is not resolved at the time of the complaint by staff present

114. Which of the following personality disorders has "cluster C" characteristics?

a. Borderline personality disorder
b. Obsessive-compulsive disorder
c. Paranoid personality disorder
d. Narcissistic personality disorder

115. Which of the following "clusters" of personality disorders has the traits of being anxious and fearful?

    a. Cluster A
    b. Cluster B
    c. Cluster C
    d. Cluster D

116. Histrionic personality disorder is defined in the DSM-5-TR as a pervasive pattern of excessive emotionality and attention seeking, beginning by early adulthood and present in a variety of contexts. An individual must possess five (or more) defined characteristics to meet the criteria for the diagnosis. Which of the following is NOT a characteristic of histrionic personality disorder?

    a. Considers relationships to be more intimate than they actually are.
    b. Believes that he or she is special and unique and can only be understood by, or should associate with, other special or high-status people.
    c. The patient is uncomfortable in situations in which he or she is not the center of attention.
    d. Displays rapidly shifting and shallow expression of emotions.

117. Being inhibited in new interpersonal situations because of feelings of inadequacy is a diagnostic criterion for which of the following personality disorders?

    a. Paranoid
    b. Dependent
    c. Antisocial
    d. Avoidant

118. Which of the following is an appropriate treatment option for antisocial personality disorder?

    a. Psychodynamic therapy
    b. Anticonvulsant medication
    c. Cognitive behavioral therapy
    d. Antidepressant medication

119. Which of the following is not an appropriate treatment goal for a patient being treated with cognitive behavioral therapy for binge eating disorder?

    a. Reducing body image concerns
    b. Reducing a patient's body mass index
    c. Reducing the symptoms of other co-morbid disorders such as anxiety or depression
    d. Reducing binge eating episodes

120. Which of the following statements accurately reflects recommendations for cognitive behavioral therapy in patients with binge eating disorder?

    a. Therapy is provided on an individual basis.
    b. Sessions are typically 30 minutes in length.
    c. A course of treatment typically includes 20 sessions.
    d. Sessions usually continue for a 12-month period.

121. Which of the following statements is NOT true regarding psychogenic non-epileptic seizures?

a. Psychogenic nonepileptic seizures most commonly present in the third decade of life.
b. Psychogenic nonepileptic seizures are seen more commonly in females.
c. Psychogenic nonepileptic seizures are often infrequent.
d. Unresponsive behavior with associated motor manifestations that may mimic a complex partial seizure or convulsion is the most common manifestation of a psychogenic nonepileptic seizure.

122. Visual hallucinations are common in patients with Lewy body dementia and Parkinson's disease. Which of the following statements best describes visual hallucinations in neurodegenerative disease?

a. In Lewy body dementia and Parkinson's disease, visual hallucinations are characteristically complex.
b. In Parkinson's disease, visual hallucinations are more prevalent earlier in the disease course.
c. In Lewy body dementia and Parkinson's disease, visual hallucinations are characteristically monocular.
d. In Lewy body dementia, visual hallucinations occur in approximately two-thirds of patients and occur late in the disease course.

123. According to the Centers for Medicare and Medicaid Services (CMS) definition of a restraint, which of the following would not meet the definition of a restraint?

a. Positioning a patient's bed sheets so tightly that the patient cannot move
b. Using side rails to prevent a patient from voluntarily getting out of bed
c. The use of a "freedom" splint to immobilize a patient's limb
d. None of the above

124. According to the Centers for Medicare and Medicaid Services (CMS), a medication may be considered a restraint when it is used as a restriction to manage a patient's behavior or restrict a patient's movement and is not a standard treatment or dosage for a patient's condition. Which of the following examples would classify a medication being utilized as a restraint?

a. A postoperative patient is administered a dose of intravenous Morphine followed by oral promethazine for complaints of pain and nausea.
b. A patient diagnosed with sleep onset insomnia is administered a benzodiazepine to assist with falling asleep.
c. A patient with dementia who is experiencing agitation and anxiety is administered a high dose of a sedative to sedate the patient and keep them in bed.
d. A patient undergoing an MRI is administered a benzodiazepine for anxiety.

125. A patient is acutely agitated and exhibiting violent behavior. Treatment with benzodiazepines and antipsychotics has not been effective for this patient and the PMHNP is considering the use of ketamine to treat his agitation. Which of the following statements is true regarding the use of ketamine for acute agitation?

a. Ketamine can exacerbate schizophrenia and should be avoided in this patient population.
b. The initial recommended dosage of ketamine is 4-5 mg/kg intravenously.
c. Notable side effects of ketamine include hypotension and bradycardia.
d. Respiratory complications are common with the use of ketamine.

126. A mental health nurse practitioner is assisting a colleague in teaching a class on managing the violent patient. Which of the following strategies might be included when teaching a clinician how to defend against assault?

    a. Avoid sudden movements and adopt a non-threatening posture if threatened with a weapon.
    b. If bitten, do not pull away rather push in towards the mouth.
    c. Maintain a sideward posture.
    d. All of the above should be included.

127. Which of the following is not a measure set that is included in the hospital based inpatient psychiatric services (HBIPS) core measures?

    a. Hours of physical restraint use
    b. Alcohol use screening
    c. Patients discharged on multiple antipsychotic medications with appropriate justification
    d. Hours of seclusion

128. An inpatient psychiatric unit's nurse practitioner knows that in order to be in compliance with the hospital based inpatient psychiatric services core measure set (specifically HBIPS-1) that the admission screening must include violence risk, substance use, and history of psychological trauma. Which additional item must also be included in the admission screening?

    a. Patient strengths
    b. Suicide risk
    c. Comorbidities
    d. Family history

129. Which of the following strategies would best support building a just culture into an organization's policies and practices?

    a. Creation of a human resource policy that authorizes punishment after a certain amount of errors
    b. Conducting educational sessions on just culture for front line staff
    c. Providing a "lessons learned" type of forum that allows staff to present actual adverse events to their peers along with ideas on how these events will be prevented from reoccurring
    d. Including language in a critical incident review policy that states that only systems will be analyzed to determine a cause of an event not human behavior

130. Behavioral theories on anxiety focus on:

    a. Classical conditioning
    b. Unresolved conflicts
    c. Social learning
    d. A and C

131. Hyperactivity of which region of the brain distinguishes obsessive convulsive disorder from other anxiety disorders?

    a. Orbitofrontal cortex
    b. Striatal regions
    c. Anterior cingulate cortex
    d. All of the above

132. Which of the following is NOT true regarding eye movement desensitization and reprocessing (EMDR)?

    a. EMDR has been widely studied and utilized as a treatment option in major depression.

    b. EMDR combines imaginal exposure and cognitive restricting with saccadic eye movements.

    c. Saccadic eye movements are induced as the client follows the therapist's rhythmic finger movements.

    d. A typical EMDR session lasts from 60-90 minutes.

133. Which of the following statements is true regarding anxiety and the geriatric population?

    a. New-onset panic attacks are common in the geriatric patient.

    b. Panic disorder is the most common anxiety disorder in geriatric patients.

    c. Geriatric patients may express anxiety symptoms as somatic symptoms.

    d. Anxiety disorders tend to decline with age.

134. The sudden onset of obsessive-compulsive symptoms in a pediatric patient may be connected to which medical etiology?

    a. Dehydration

    b. Streptococcal infection

    c. Gastroenteritis

    d. Anemia

135. A ten-year-old patient was just diagnosed with pediatric autoimmune neuropsychiatric disorder associated with streptococcal infections (PANDAS). Which of the following symptoms (in addition to obsessive compulsive disorder symptoms) is not commonly associated with PANDAS?

    a. Urinary urgency

    b. Joint pain

    c. Sleep disturbances

    d. Hyperactivity

136. Which of the following is NOT a risk factor for the development of postpartum psychosis?

    a. History of bipolar disorder

    b. Recent discontinuation of lithium

    c. Family history of postpartum psychosis

    d. Multiparity

137. Which of the following is NOT a typical neurologic manifestation of Wilson's disease?

    a. Dysarthria

    b. Drooling

    c. Hyporeflexia

    d. Dystonia

138. Which of the following neurologic manifestations is the most common in patients with neurologic Wilson's disease?

    a. Parkinsonism
    b. Dysarthria
    c. Myoclonia
    d. Tremors

139. Kayser-Fleischer rings are brownish or gray-green rings that are caused by fine, pigmented, granular deposits of copper in the cornea. Which of the following neurologic diseases are Kayser-Fleischer rings likely to be found?

    a. Huntington's disease
    b. Parkinson's disease
    c. Lewy body dementia
    d. Wilson's disease

140. Which of the following statements is NOT true regarding photic-induced seizures?

    a. Photo-convulsive seizures are usually focal; however, they may be generalized.
    b. Children are more susceptible to photic-induced seizures than adults.
    c. A propensity for photic-induced seizures may be inherited.
    d. Individuals may be sensitive to certain light triggers but not others.

141. Which of the following best describes the type of electrode placement used in electroconvulsive therapy that has the greatest efficacy in treating depression?

    a. Bifrontal
    b. Right unilateral
    c. Bilateral
    d. Left unilateral

142. All of the following are potential physiologic effects of alcohol toxicity EXCEPT:

    a. Leukocytosis
    b. Gastric ulceration
    c. Peripheral neuropathy
    d. Hepatitis

143. A patient with Wernicke-Korsakoff syndrome may present with which of the following sets of symptoms?

    a. Arrhythmias, chest pain, ischemic colitis, and seizures
    b. Nystagmus, ataxia, paralysis of ocular muscles, and somnolence
    c. Hypoglycemia, thrombocytopenia, somnolence, and elevated serum ammonia
    d. Nausea, abdominal cramping, body aches, and anxiety

144. The American Society of Addiction Medicine's Patient Placement Criteria (ASAM PPC-2R) defines substance abuse treatment on a continuum that contains five levels of care. Which of the following is considered to be level 2 on the continuum?

    a. Early intervention
    b. Residential/inpatient treatment
    c. Outpatient treatment
    d. Intensive outpatient/partial hospitalization treatment

145. Which of the following best describes the recommended dosing schedule for thiamine in the use of alcohol intoxication/withdrawal?

a. Thiamine, 50 mg IM/IV for three days, followed by 100 mg P.O. twice daily
b. Thiamine, 200 mg IM/IV for three days, followed by 100 mg P.O. twice daily
c. Thiamine, 100 mg IM/IV daily, or 100 mg P.O. three times daily for three days, followed by 100 mg P.O. daily
d. Thiamine, 100 mg IV daily for five days, followed by 200 mg P.O. daily

146. Which of the following statements is NOT true regarding the use of Librium in the treatment of alcohol intoxication/withdrawal?

a. Librium has a long half-life.
b. Librium is metabolized by the liver.
c. Librium is best absorbed intramuscularly.
d. Librium can be tapered up for worsening alcohol withdrawal symptoms or down to lessen sedation.

147. Which of the following is a contraindication in the use of disulfiram as a deterrent to alcohol use?

a. Liver disease
b. Working in a factory where fumes are inhaled
c. Being a carrier of viral hepatitis
d. All of the above

148. Which of the following agents used in the treatment of alcohol addiction is available in depo form and administered as a monthly injection?

a. Buprenorphine
b. Naltrexone
c. Acamprosate
d. Disulfiram

149. It is recommended that the first day dose of methadone for treatment of opioid dependence/withdrawal not exceed what dosage?

a. 20 mg
b. 30 mg
c. 40 mg
d. 50 mg

150. Which of the following is included in the eligibility criteria (according to federal regulations) for a patient to be placed on a methadone maintenance program?

a. Documentation of the presence of an opioid use disorder for at least one year of continuous use
b. An age of 21 or older
c. Pregnancy along with the presence of an opioid use disorder for at least one year of continuous use
d. Documented attendance at counseling sessions

151. Which of the following statements is NOT true regarding buprenorphine?

    a. A hospitalized patient may be treated with buprenorphine by a clinician without a DEA waiver.

    b. Clinicians providing office-based buprenorphine must specify that they have capacity to provide or refer patients for counseling.

    c. Buprenorphine is a class II substance.

    d. Induction with buprenorphine may be performed in a clinician's office under observation or in the patient's home setting.

152. Which of the following medications is most recommended in the treatment of patients with moderate to severe opioid use disorder?

    a. Levo-alpha-acetylmethadol

    b. Naltrexone

    c. Buprenorphine

    d. Methadone

153. Methadone has the potential to increase the QTc interval and may cause torsades de pointes. As a result, the FDA issued a black-box warning in 2006 to alert clinicians of this potential. Which of the following strategies should be implemented prior to starting a patient on methadone given this warning?

    a. Obtain a baseline echocardiogram prior to initiation of methadone.

    b. Assess the patient for other risk factors for QTc prolongation.

    c. Begin the patient on oral magnesium sulfate in conjunction with the methadone.

    d. Methadone should not be considered for use in patients with a QTc interval greater than 450 msec.

154. According to the Centers for Medicare and Medicaid (CMS), in which of the following circumstances would one NOT report a death associated with restraint or seclusion?

    a. A death that occurred while a patient was in restraints but not seclusion and the only restraints used on the patient were applied exclusively to the patient's wrist(s) and were composed solely of soft, non-rigid, cloth-like materials.

    b. A death known to the hospital that occurred within one week after restraint or seclusion where it is reasonable to assume that use of restraint or placement in seclusion contributed directly or indirectly to the patient's death, regardless of the type(s) of restraint used on the patient during this time.

    c. A death that occurred within 24 hours after the patient had been removed from restraint or seclusion, excluding those in which only 2-point soft wrist restraints were used and the patient was not in seclusion within 24 hours of their death

    d. A death that occurred while a patient is in restraint or seclusion, excluding those in which only 2-point soft wrist restraints were used and the patient was not in seclusion at the time of death

155. According to the Centers for Medicare and Medicaid (CMS) Conditions of Participation (482.13 (f) (1)), staff must be trained and able to demonstrate competency in restraints, including the application, monitoring, assessment, and provision of care for patients in restraints:

   a. Before performing any clinical interventions (specified in 482.13 (f) (1)) related to restraints
   b. As part of orientation
   c. Consistent with frequency outlined in hospital policy
   d. In all of the above scenarios

156. Which of the following disorders is defined as a motor-behavioral condition that occurs from genetic mutations for the coding of the enzyme hypoxanthine-guanine phosphoribosyltransferase (HPRT) resulting in hyperuricemia?

   a. Benign hereditary chorea
   b. Lesch-Nyhan syndrome
   c. ADCY5-related dyskinesia
   d. Rett syndrome

157. Which of the following statements is not true regarding stereotypies in children?

   a. Rett syndrome is an example of a disorder characterized by marked stereotypies.
   b. Lower extremities are typically not involved.
   c. They only occur in children with developmental disorders.
   d. They may include repetitive chewing, rocking, tapping, twirling, or touching.

158. Sydenham chorea is associated with which psychiatric disorder?

   a. Major depression
   b. Bipolar disorder
   c. Schizophrenia
   d. Obsessive-compulsive disorder

159. Which of the following classifications of medications has the potential to cause chorea?

   a. Anticonvulsants
   b. Central nervous system stimulants
   c. Calcium channel blockers
   d. All of the above

160. Which of the following statements is true regarding tardive dyskinesia?

   a. Tardive dyskinesia is much less common in children than adults.
   b. Tardive dyskinesia is irreversible.
   c. Tardive dyskinesia typically appears 1-2 years after antipsychotic treatment is initiated.
   d. It is common for tardive dyskinesia to first appear after an increase in dose.

161. Which of the following practitioners can complete the one hour face-to-face assessment of a patient restrained for the management of violent or self-destructive behavior according to the Centers for Medicare and Medicaid?

   a. A physician
   b. A physician or physician extender (APN, PA)
   c. A registered nurse
   d. All of the above

162. Tardive dystonia is defined as:

a. Tachypnea, irregular breathing rhythms, and grunting noises

b. Limited to a relatively short period of time during the course of treatment with antipsychotic drugs followed by spontaneous resolution

c. Tardive dyskinesia in which more sustained dystonic manifestations predominate

d. Late-appearing motor restlessness

163. Which of the following symptoms is likely to be seen in a patient diagnosed with neuroferritinopathy?

a. Dystonia, myoclonus, and peripheral neuropathy

b. Seizures, myopathy, and behavioral changes

c. Parkinsonism, dystonia, and cognitive decline

d. Intellectually disabled, self-mutilating behavior, and developmental delays

164. Which of the following diagnostic tests is recommended for a patient presenting to the emergency department with new-onset seizures?

a. Functional MRI (fMRI)

b. Computed tomography (CT)

c. Positron emission tomography (PET)

d. Magnetic resonance imaging (MRI)

165. Which of the following variants of primary progressive aphasia is characterized by impaired single-word retrieval along with repetition with errors in speech and naming with spared single-word comprehension, motor speech, and object knowledge?

a. Agrammatism

b. Semantic

c. Logopenic

d. Nonfluent

166. Which of the following statements is true regarding attention deficit hyperactivity disorder in adults versus children?

a. Symptoms of hyperactivity or impulsivity are more obvious or overt in adults.

b. Attention deficit hyperactivity disorder in children rarely continues into adulthood.

c. Symptoms of inattention are less prominent in adults.

d. Other psychiatric disorders may occur in conjunction with attention deficit hyperactivity disorder in adults, including mood and anxiety disorders, substance use disorder, and intermittent explosive disorder.

167. Which of the following is a manifestation of executive dysfunction in adult patients with attention deficit hyperactivity disorder?

a. Mood lability

b. Deficit in self-monitoring

c. Restlessness

d. Motivational deficits

168. Which of the following best describes the recommended indications for assertive community treatment?

    a. Individuals with severe mental illness who wish to work

    b. Individuals with major depression that wish to utilize a treatment alternative to antidepressant medications

    c. Individuals with moderate to severe mental illness that are in need of pre and post-discharge coordination

    d. Individuals with severe mental illness with a recent history of repeated hospitalization or homelessness

169. Which of the following statements is not true regarding the use of ketamine in conjunction with electroconvulsive therapy (ECT)?

    a. Ketamine can prolong ECT seizures.

    b. Ketamine can cause hypotension in higher doses.

    c. Post-ECT disorientation can occur when ketamine is used for induction of anesthesia prior to ECT treatment.

    d. Ketamine appears to initially enhance the benefits of ECT.

170. Which of the following is not an indication for electroconvulsive therapy (ECT)?

    a. Delirium

    b. Schizophrenia

    c. Adjustment disorder with depressed mood

    d. Severe unipolar depression

171. Which of the following legislative acts authorized funding to train participants in the recognition of symptoms of mental illness and substance abuse?

    a. Mental Health Reform Act of 2015

    b. Helping Families in Mental Health Crisis Act

    c. The Mental Health First Aid Act of 2015

    d. The Mental Health Study Act

172. According to Hildegard Peplau's theory of interpersonal relations, which of the following "roles of the nurse" is defined as "one who provides a specific needed information that aids in the understanding of a problem or new situation?"

    a. Leader

    b. Resource person

    c. Counselor

    d. Teacher

173. In which phase of the interpersonal relationship according to Peplau's theory of interpersonal relations would a client make full use of services offered?

    a. Resolution phase

    b. Identification phase

    c. Exploitation phase

    d. Orientation phase

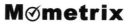

174. Hildegard Peplau defines four levels of anxiety in her theory of interpersonal relations. Which level of anxiety involves feelings of dread and terror in which a person cannot be redirected to a task?

    a. Panic
    b. Severe
    c. Mild
    d. Moderate

175. Which of the following statements is not true regarding Hildegard Peplau's theory of interpersonal relations?

    a. The concepts in this theory are applicable only to mental health patients.
    b. The phases of the therapeutic nurse-client are highly comparable to the nursing process.
    c. Health promotion and maintenance are less emphasized in this theory.
    d. The theory includes four phases of the nurse-client relationship.

Answers and Explanations

1. C: The concepts of transference, counter transference and defense mechanisms are components of psychodynamic theories. Sigmund Freud, Carl Jung, and Alfred Adler are well known for their development of psychodynamic theories. The basic premise of psychodynamic theory is that there are conscious and unconscious mental processes that guide and influence a person's thought and behavior. The focus of psychodynamic therapy is the unconscious processes and how they relate to and affect a person's behavior.

2. D: Acceptance is not a component of the transtheoretical model of behavior. This model of behavior change is most commonly used in health behavior change research and practice. The core concepts of this model include stages of change, processes of change, self-efficacy, and decisional balance. In this model, an individual works through each stage in an attempt to make personal changes in his or her life. The stages include: pre-contemplation, contemplation, preparation, action, maintenance, and termination.

3. B: In the transtheoretical model of behavior change, a client works through a series of stages in an attempt to make a personal change. In the maintenance stage, the individual is actively working to prevent a relapse in the problematic behavior. A client remains in the maintenance stage as long as the problematic behavior no longer occurs. In the termination stage, the individual no longer has the temptation to continue the problematic behavior and has confidence that the behavior will never occur again. In the preparation stage, the individual begins to plan taking action on eliminating the problematic behavior and may take small steps to work toward change. In the contemplation stage, the individual begins to have some awareness that the behavior is problematic and begins to consider both the pros and cons of changing the behavior.

4. D: Hildegard Peplau developed her theory of interpersonal relationships in the 1950's and is considered to be the founder of psychiatric nursing. Peplau's theory of interpersonal relationships is a middle range descriptive classification theory that states a person is a developing self-system composed of biochemical, physiological, and interpersonal characteristics and needs. Peplau proposed that anxiety is produced when an individual is in some way threatened. The nurse's role in Peplau's theory is to assist the client in understanding their anxiety and utilize different behaviors in an attempt to use the anxiety to affect a positive outcome.

5. A: The PICO model is a commonly used tool used to guide clinicians in utilizing evidence-based practice. The model consists of the following components: P: Who is the patient population? I: What is the potential intervention? C: Is there a comparison intervention or control group? O: What is the desired outcome? This model can be used by clinicians to guide their evidence-based practice projects to ensure the relevancy of the project and a thorough evaluation of the evidence prior to adoption of the evidence into practice.

6. C: The next step in the evidence-based practice process would be the assessment of the current practice using patient specific scenarios to frame the clinical question. The clinical question should be searchable and answerable. Clinical questions should take into consideration the population, intervention or topic of interest, comparison and intervention groups, outcomes, and time.

7. B: Personal experience is not a key component of evidence-based practice. Evidence based practice is defined as the integration of best research evidence, clinical expertise, and patient values to guide clinical care. Key components of evidence-based practice include clinical expertise, patient values and preferences and current research evidence. Research evidence may include qualitative and outcomes research and clinical trials. Clinical expertise may include knowledge gained from healthcare experience.

8. C: Nurse theorist Laura Polk worked to develop a middle range theory of resilience in nursing in the late 1990's. Resiliency is defined as the ability to transform a disastrous situation into a growth experience in an effort to move forward. Self-efficacy is defined as one's belief in one's ability to succeed in specific situations. Concordance is defined as a way of working together with people. Adaptation is defined as an individual's ability to adjust to changes and new or different experiences.

9. B: Concordance is a way of working with others and may be used in the healthcare setting to develop a mutually agreed upon treatment plan between a health care provider and a patient. Adherence is the process of staying with a course of treatment. Compliance is the process of following a set of instructions. Patient centered care is defined as a method of providing care that is considerate of individual patient preferences, needs and values and ensuring that those values help to guide clinical decisions.

10. A: The clinical skills/professional behaviors of a clinician that focus on the cultural beliefs, values, and perceptions of the patient during the therapeutic relationship established between the patient and clinician. Culturally competent care includes the recognition of an individual's cultural beliefs, values, and perceptions. According to nurse theorist Madeleine Leininger, culturally competent healthcare providers possess the clinical skills and professional behaviors that allow them to assist and support their patients in retaining and/or preserving relevant care values so that they may maintain well-being and recover from illness. Culture is defined as a way of life belonging to an individual or group of individuals that reflects values and customs. Diversity is the recognition that each individual is unique along the dimensions of race, gender, ethnicity, religious beliefs, and sexual orientation. Cultural appropriation is the adoption of the elements of one culture by members of a different culture.

11. D: Acetylcholine is not an example of a monoamine neurotransmitter. There are over 100 different neurotransmitters known to exist in the human brain. Amines, amino acids, neuropeptides, and circulating hormones are common types of neurotransmitters. Dopamine, serotonin, epinephrine, and norepinephrine are monoamine neurotransmitters. Monoamine neurotransmitters are derived from amino acids. The decarboxylase enzyme removes the carboxylic acid from their structure, thereby removing the "acid."

12. C: The neurotransmitter serotonin is derived from the amino acid tryptophan and is synthesized in the raphe nuclei of the brain stem. Serotonin is implicated in the regulation of sleep, mood, pain, and appetite. The physiologic effects of an increase in the adrenergic neurotransmitter norepinephrine include tachycardia, hypertension, vasoconstriction, anxiety, and hyperactivity. Glutamate is an excitatory neurotransmitter necessary for learning and memory. Gamma-aminobutyric acid is a potent inhibitory neurotransmitter that has an effect on motor control and vision. It also regulates anxiety.

13. B: A medication that works as a neurotransmitter's agonist mimics the neurotransmitter and has the same effect on the postsynaptic neuron as the neurotransmitter. An antagonist is a molecule that blocks the effect of the neurotransmitter on the post-synaptic neuron. A synapse is the microscopic gap between neurons. A membrane receptor is a large protein attached to the cell membrane of the post-synaptic neuron.

14. B: Catecholamines are derived from the amino acid tyrosine and are synthesized in the brain, adrenal medulla and by some sympathetic nerve fibers. Dopamine, norepinephrine, and epinephrine are all catecholamines, characterized by a catechol group attached to an amine. Catecholamines play a role in nutrient metabolism, thermogenesis, glycogenolysis, and hormone secretion.

15. D: Antipsychotics are differentiated by potency and are classified as low, moderate, or high potency. If an antipsychotic medication is classified as high potency, a smaller dose is needed to achieve the intended response. The high potency antipsychotics include haloperidol and fluphenazine. These medications are associated with a higher incidence of extrapyramidal side effects. Loxapine and Perphenazine are classified as moderate potency antipsychotics. Low potency antipsychotics include chlorpromazine and thioridazine. These medications have a higher potency for cholinergic and alpha-1 adrenergic receptors and therefore are associated with a higher incidence of anticholinergic side effects.

16. C: Neuroleptic malignant syndrome (NMS) is a rare, life-threatening neurologic emergency that may occur in patients taking neuroleptic agents such as haloperidol and fluphenazine. Although NMS is more commonly seen in patients taking higher potency antipsychotics, lower potency antipsychotics and newer "atypical" antipsychotics have also been implicated in this condition. NMS is characterized by acute onset (over 1-3 days) development of symptoms including mental status changes, hyperthermia, muscular rigidity, diaphoresis, tachycardia, labile blood pressure, and dysrhythmias. Laboratory findings commonly include an elevated serum creatine phosphokinase and an elevated white blood cell count as well as electrolyte abnormalities.

17. D: The use of dantrolene may be considered in patients with neuroleptic malignant syndrome that do not respond to the discontinuation of the neuroleptic agent and supportive care within the first day or two of treatment. Dantrolene appears to shorten the duration of the illness and reduce body temperature and muscle rigidity. It is used in the treatment of malignant hyperthermia. Antimuscarinic agents such as benztropine and atropine are not recommended in the treatment of neuroleptic malignant syndrome. Chlorpromazine is an antipsychotic that should be immediately discontinued in patients with neuroleptic malignant syndrome.

18. A: Malignant catatonia is a type of catatonia that is characterized by an inability to move normally. It can occur in patients with underlying psychiatric disorders as well as patients with general medical disorders. Common symptoms associated with catatonia include immobility, posturing, stupor, negativism, staring and echolalia. Malignant catatonia can also share the clinical features of hyperthermia and rigidity with neuroleptic malignant syndrome, making it difficult to differentiate between the two conditions.

19. C: Decreased bowel sounds are not a common physical finding in selective serotonin syndrome. Selective serotonin syndrome is a syndrome that occurs with increased serotonergic activity of the central nervous system. It can potentially be life-threatening and is characterized by mental status changes as well as neuromuscular alterations /abnormalities. Common physical findings include hyperthermia, rigidity, agitation, akathisia, tremor, dry mucus membranes, increased bowel sounds, dilated pupils, and hyperreflexia. Neuromuscular symptoms are more commonly experienced in the lower extremities. Hypertension and tachycardia are also common physical findings.

20. C: The antidote cyproheptadine is a histamine-1 receptor antagonist that may be used in the treatment of patients with selective serotonin syndrome when the administration of benzodiazepines and supportive therapy are ineffective. Treatment with bromocriptine, propranolol and dantrolene is not recommended. Propranolol may cause prolonged hypotension and has the potential to mask tachycardia. The use of dantrolene has not been proven effective in the treatment of patients with selective serotonin syndrome. Bromocriptine is a serotonin agonist contraindicated in the treatment of serotonin syndrome as it may exacerbate the syndrome.

21. A: Criteria for a diagnosis of catatonia are met when the clinical presentation is dominated by at least three of the following criteria: stupor, catalepsy, wavy flexibility, mutism, negativism, posturing, mannerisms, stereotypy, agitation or excessive motor activity, grimacing, echolalia, and echopraxia. Akathisia (excessive, uncontrolled fidgeting) is not part of the clinical criteria used to define catatonia. Psychiatric diagnoses of bipolar disorders, major depression, psychotic disorders, and autistic spectrum disorders may include the presence of the behavioral syndrome catatonia.

22. B: There are no specific laboratory tests used in the diagnosis of catatonia, however in malignant catatonia the white blood cell count may be elevated (15,000-25,000/mL), creatinine kinase may be elevated (levels exceeding 1000 IU/L are strongly correlated with malignant catatonia) and the serum iron level may be decreased (can occur in up to 40% of patients with malignant catatonia). Serum bicarbonate levels are not affected by malignant catatonia but may be decreased in patients with selective serotonin syndrome.

23. C: The three principal subtypes of catatonia include excited catatonia, retarded catatonia, and malignant catatonia. In retarded catatonia, common signs and symptoms include staring, posturing, mutism, inhibited movement, and negativism. Speech and spontaneous movement may be reduced and in severe cases stupor may occur. Excited catatonia is characterized by hyperkinesis, restlessness, frenzy, and combativeness. Delirium may also occur in severe cases. Malignant catatonia is a potentially life-threatening condition characterized by fever, delirium, rigidity, and autonomic instability. The symptoms of malignant catatonia may also mimic those of neuroleptic malignant syndrome.

24. A: Recommended first line pharmacologic therapy for bipolar patients that present with acute hypomania or mild to moderate manic symptoms includes risperidone or olanzapine as monotherapy. Other pharmacologic agents proven effective include haloperidol, cariprazine, lithium, carbamazepine, paliperidone, aripiprazole, asenapine, quetiapine, ziprasidone, and valproate. Lithium in combination with valproate is a treatment option in patients with hypomania or mild to moderate mania that have not responded to three to five monotherapy trials. Ziprasidone is generally recommended to be avoided as adjunctive therapy in first line medication combinations for the treatment of bipolar disorder. Lamotrigine was not proven to be effective (when compared to placebo) in the treatment of hypomania or mild to moderate mania.

25. D: Life-threatening adverse reactions including Stevens-Johnson syndrome and toxic epidermal necrolysis may occur with the administration of carbamazepine, most commonly in the first eight weeks of therapy. Stevens-Johnson syndrome is a rare disorder that is characterized by the development of flu-like symptoms followed by the formation of a reddish/purplish skin rash that rapidly spreads, causing blistering and shedding of the skin. This type of reaction occurs most commonly (up to 5% of patients) in patients with the HLA-B*1502 allele. This allele is most commonly found in patients of Asian descent including South Asian Indians. The U.S. FDA recommends that screening for this allele be conducted prior to the initiation of carbamazepine in patients of Asian or South Asian Indian descent.

26. B: The statement, "I should continue taking my Ativan prior to my ECT treatment" requires further education. Electroconvulsive therapy treatments cause chemical changes in the brain that help to relieve severe depression. Patients should be instructed that multiple ECT treatments may be necessary and the number of treatments is dependent on the patient's response to therapy.

Patient education should include informing the patient that he or she may feel confused after waking up from the ECT treatment. Patients are instructed to take any anti-hypertensive medications that they are currently taking with a small sip of water approximately 2 hours prior to the procedure. Benzodiazepines should be tapered and discontinued when possible for patients undergoing ECT treatment. Benzodiazepines can increase seizure threshold, shorten seizure duration, and decrease the intensity of the ECT seizure, thereby decreasing the efficacy of the ECT treatment. In patients that cannot tolerate discontinuation of their benzodiazepine, the evening dose of the benzodiazepine can be held the evening prior to the scheduled ECT treatment.

27. D: Lithium toxicity may be acute, acute on chronic, or chronic in nature. Signs and symptoms of lithium toxicity are dependent upon the rate of onset as well as the overall total body burden of the lithium. Signs and symptoms may include nausea, vomiting, diarrhea, prolonged QTc interval, bradycardia, sluggishness, ataxia, confusion, tremors, and agitation. In severe cases, seizures and encephalopathy can occur. Lithium toxicity is not associated with an elevation in cardiac biomarkers.

28. B: Lithium therapy is normally initiated at a starting dose of 300 milligrams to be administered 2-3 times daily and then increased by 300-600 milligrams every 1-5 days depending on the patient's tolerance, body mass index and overall response. The recommended therapeutic concentration of lithium is 0.8-1.2 mEq/L, not to exceed 1.2mEq/L. The therapeutic serum level is usually achieved with a daily dose of 900-1800 milligrams of lithium. Patients that cannot tolerate a 0.8 mEq/L serum level may respond to a 0.6 mEq/L serum level.

29. D: "I know I need to watch my salt intake. I have recently been eating foods with a higher amount of sodium." Serum lithium levels are affected by renal function as well as sodium and water balance. Dehydration (may occur with high fever or gastrointestinal illness), decreased sodium intake and impaired renal function all have the potential to increase serum lithium levels. Conversely, increased sodium intake causes increased sodium and lithium excretion, thereby potentially decreasing the serum lithium level.

30. D: There are many different medications that have the potential to interact with lithium. Patients taking these medications should have lithium levels closely monitored. Medications with the potential to interact with lithium and increase serum lithium levels include non-steroidal anti-inflammatory medications, thiazide diuretics, angiotensin converting enzyme (ACE) inhibitors, metronidazole, and tetracycline antibiotics. Potassium sparing diuretics and theophylline have the potential to decrease the serum lithium level.

31. C: Both psychotherapy and pharmacotherapy affect the corticolimbic pathway of the brain. They differ in the specific sites that they target. Psychotherapy is believed to affect the prefrontal cortex by enhancing its function and then down to the limbic system in a top-down manner. Conversely, pharmacotherapy is believed to first target the limbic system and then work its way up to the prefrontal cortex in a bottom down manner.

32. C: Omega-3 fatty acids are nutrients found primarily in fish and seafood. Omega-3 supplements from fish oil may be used as a complementary therapy/adjunctive treatment for patients with mood disorders. Omega-3 fatty acids work by increasing serotonin levels, altering dopamine function, and regulating corticotrophin-releasing factor. The usual dose is 1.0-9.6 g/day. Side effects are usually minimal but may include gastrointestinal disturbances and alteration in glucose metabolism in patients with diabetes.

33. D: Valerian is an herb known for its calming effects. It works by inhibiting the enzymes responsible for breaking down GABA. 400-800 mg of valerian root may be taken 2 hours before bedtime to enhance sleep. Side effects include gastrointestinal disturbances, restlessness, headache and rebound anxiety (if abruptly discontinued). Valerian may also cause additive effects with alcohol, benzodiazepines, and other sedatives.

34. C: Cognitive side effects of transcranial magnetic stimulation are similar to those experienced in ECT treatment. Transcranial magnetic stimulation (TMS) is an alternate treatment option to antidepressant therapy in patients with mood disorders. TMS is an outpatient procedure that utilizes similar technology as magnetic resonance imaging (MRI). There are no cognitive side effects like those experienced with ECT treatment. The patient is awake during the procedure as it does not require any medication or anesthesia. The treatment takes less than 1 hour and is typically administered daily over 4-6 weeks. Treatment is expensive and often not reimbursed by insurance companies.

35. C: Medically refractory partial onset seizures also utilize vagal nerve stimulation for treatment. Vagal nerve stimulation (VNS) treatment involves the surgical implantation of a pulse generating device with a wire attached to the left vagus nerve. The incoming sensory connections of the vagus nerve are directly connected to the parts of the brain affected by psychiatric disorders. Side effects of VNS treatment include hoarseness, cough, and mild shortness of breath. VNS is not widely used in the treatment of depression due to the high cost of treatment, limited reimbursement by insurance companies, and minimal effectiveness in the treatment of depression. VNS is currently being studied for effectiveness in multiple sclerosis, headaches, pain, and Alzheimer's disease. It is more commonly used as a treatment option for patients with medically refractory partial onset seizures.

36. A: Cranial nerve VII is the nerve associated with facial expression. Anticholinergic effects associated with this cranial nerve include dry mouth, decreased respiratory secretions, and decreased tearing. Cranial nerve III is the oculomotor nerve. Anticholinergic effects associated with this cranial nerve include mydriasis and blurred vision. Cranial nerve IX is the glossopharyngeal nerve. Anticholinergic effects associated with this cranial nerve include dry mouth and decreased respiratory secretions. Cranial nerve X is the vagus nerve. Anticholinergic effects associated with this cranial nerve include constipation, urinary hesitancy, and increased heart rate.

37. D: Fluoxetine is the most studied selective serotonin reuptake inhibitor in the treatment of bulimia nervosa and the only U.S. FDA approved antidepressant for the treatment of bulimia nervosa. Sertraline has been shown to be effective in the decreasing of symptoms associated with bulimia nervosa including depression, anxiety, and obsessive-compulsive behaviors. Phenelzine, isocarboxazid, brofaromine, lithium, phenytoin, carbamazepine, and topiramate have also shown improvement in treating the symptoms of bulimia nervosa.

38. B: Hyperkalemia is not a characteristic of re-feeding syndrome. Re-feeding syndrome is a rare but life-threatening condition that can occur when reintroducing food to a person who has experienced significant weight loss. Re-feeding syndrome is characterized by electrolyte and fluid imbalance including the potential for hypophosphatemia, hypomagnesemia, hypokalemia, glucose intolerance, thiamine deficiency, and fluid overload.

39. C: Anorexia nervosa is a psychiatric disorder characterized by a refusal to maintain a healthy body weigh combined with an obsessive fear of gaining weight. Anorexia nervosa is ten times more prevalent in females than males and typically begins in adolescence. It carries the highest death rate (over 5%) of all the psychiatric disorders. It is often underdiagnosed and undertreated as many affected by anorexia do not seek treatment.

40. D: Diagnostic criteria for both unipolar major depression and bipolar major depression are very similar in nature without any specific symptoms to differentiate the two. There are however some clinical features that are more commonly seen in patients with bipolar major depression. They include hypersomnia, hyperphagia, and leaden paralysis. In addition, delusions and hallucinations are more common in bipolar major depression. Social functioning is noted to be poorer in patients with bipolar major depression as opposed to unipolar major depression.

41. C: Co-morbid anxiety disorders and substance use disorders are NOT more common in the geriatric population. Clinical features of bipolar disorder differ somewhat in the geriatric patient (>50 years of age). The pathogenesis of bipolar disorder in the geriatric patient may be related to reduced volume of gray matter, hyperintensities of white matter and biochemical changes. Some of the differences in clinical features seen in the geriatric patient with bipolar disorder include cognitive impairment that is more common and severe, higher instances of co-morbid general medical disorders, lower instances of co-morbid anxiety and substance use disorders, and a lower instance of excessive sexual interest/behavior during manic/hypomanic episodes.

42. C: According to DSM-5-TR diagnostic criteria for hypomania includes a distinct period of abnormally and persistently elevated, expansive, or irritable mood and abnormally and persistently increased activity or energy, lasting at least four consecutive days and present most of the day, nearly every day. Three or more of the following symptoms must also be present: inflated self-esteem or grandiosity, decreased need for sleep, more talkative than usual or the need to keep talking, flight of ideas or racing thoughts, distractibility, increase in goal-directed activity, and excessive involvement in risky activities that have a high potential for painful consequences. When psychotic features are present, the episode is defined as manic.

43. D: There are multiple medications and substances that have the capacity to induce psychosis. Examples include analgesics, anti-depressants, antivirals, anticholinergics, corticosteroids, anabolic steroids, antiepileptics, hallucinogens, interferons, stimulants, and cannabinoids. Alcohol and toxins such as carbon monoxide and heavy metals also have the capacity to induce psychosis. Anticoagulants are not associated with the development of psychosis.

44. C: A manic episode with mixed features includes the presences of at least three of the following symptoms present for most days of the episode: depressed mood, low energy, diminished interest or pleasure in most activities, psychomotor retardation, excessive guilt or thoughts of worthlessness, and recurrent thoughts about death or suicide or a suicide attempt. Flight of ideas is associated with an episode of major depression with mixed features.

45. B: Patients with mixed features are at greater risk for suicidal ideation and behavior. Mood episodes with mixed features occur frequently, ranging from 20-70% in bipolar patients. It is uncommon for mood episodes with mixed features to transition to mania. Episodes with mixed features can evolve into major depression. Response to treatment is often poorer in mood episodes with mixed features as compared to pure mania or pure bipolar major depression.

46. B: Somatization is the process of converting psychological conflicts into bodily symptoms. It is a defense mechanism with a lower level of adaptation and maturity. Altruism is defined as constructive, gratifying service to others. Sublimation is the process of channeling instincts into socially acceptable actions. Altruism, sublimation, and humor are all defense mechanisms associated with higher adaptation and maturity.

47. D: Projection is a lower adaptive defense mechanism defined as reacting to unacceptable thoughts or impulses as if outside of oneself. Distortion is defined as reshaping external reality, for example, hallucinations or delusions. Dissociation is the absence of conscious awareness of behaviors of the coexistence of separate mental systems or identities. Intellectualization is the excessive use of intellect to avoid feelings or experiences.

48. B: Failure to thrive is infants is defined as failure to appropriately gain weight. In severe cases, failure to thrive may contribute to secondary immune deficiency, short stature and permanent damage to the brain and central nervous system. Failure to thrive in infants is characterized by weight below the 3rd percentile in body charts, iron deficiency, behavioral problems, psychomotor delay and feeding problems with no identified disease process.

49. D: There are many possible treatment options for patients with mood disorders. Treatment modalities include self-help, psychotherapy, pharmacotherapy, alternative or complementary therapy, electroconvulsive therapy, transcranial magnetic stimulation, and vagal nerve stimulation. In patients with severe depression, treatment may include the use of a selective serotonin reuptake inhibitor, psychotherapy and inpatient or partial hospitalization. If psychotic symptoms are also present, an antipsychotic may be added.

50. C: In patients with severe depression and a history of polarity, omega-3 fatty acids, mood stabilizing agents, dark therapy, social rhythm therapy, and interpersonal therapy are all recommended treatment options. Self-help (either group or individual), supportive therapy, exercise, Vitamin D, bright light, melatonin, and St. John's wort are viable treatment options in patients with mild depression.

51. D: Positive symptoms associated with schizophrenia include hallucinations (may be auditory, visual, somatic, olfactory, or gustatory), delusions, and disorganized thoughts and behavior. Positive symptoms represent an exaggeration of a normal process. Conversely, negative symptoms are the absence or diminishing of normal process. Negative symptoms may include lack of energy, apathy, and a flat affect. Negative symptoms may be classified as either primary or secondary.

52. B: Patients are NOT more likely to have a depressive disorder in deficit schizophrenia. Although not classified as a distinct DSM-5-TR subtype of schizophrenia, there are marked clinical distinctions in patients who primarily experience the negative symptoms of schizophrenia (deficit schizophrenia). Patients with deficit schizophrenia are less likely to experience delusions with a high emotional content, less likely to have a substance use disorder, less likely to have a depressive disorder, and less likely to show improvement or recover.

53. B: Neurological "soft signs" are defined as subtle impairments of motor coordination and sensory integration. Astereognosis, agraphesthesia, and right-left confusion are common deficits present in patients with schizophrenia. Astereognosis is the inability to recognize familiar objects by touch alone. Agraphesthesia is the inability to recognize letters or numbers when traced on the skin. Akathisia is defined as a subjective sense of restlessness or actual restlessness.

54. D: Hypertension, hyperlipidemia, and diabetes are all metabolic disturbances associated with schizophrenia. In regards to diabetes, there is evidence to support that patients with schizophrenia have a resistance to insulin. In addition, hypertension, hyperlipidemia, and diabetes may be linked to schizophrenia due to the presence of other risk factors commonly seen in patients with schizophrenia including a sedentary lifestyle and smoking. Life expectancy in patients with schizophrenia is reduced largely in part to the presence of heart disease.

55. C: Schizophreniform disorder, schizoaffective disorder, bipolar disorder, substance induced psychotic disorders, and major depression with psychotic features are all common psychiatric disorders in the differential diagnoses of schizophrenia. In schizophreniform disorder, all criteria for schizophrenia are met with the total duration of the disorder being less than six months. Schizoaffective disorder includes all of the features of schizophrenia with an associated mania or a significant depressive component. Major depression with psychotic features as well as bipolar disorder also include a significant mood component. In substance induced psychotic disorders, symptoms subside when the individual is sober.

56. A: When traditional therapies are ineffective in the treatment of schizophrenia, there are several strategies that should be implemented prior to deeming a patient "treatment resistant." The patient should be assessed for other causes of residual symptoms of schizophrenia. In addition, optimization of current antipsychotic drug treatment as well as non-pharmacologic interventions should be trialed prior to the initiation of a clozapine trial. Clozapine is indicated in schizophrenic patients deemed treatment resistant (patients who have trialed two antipsychotic medications at the maximum tolerated dose (within the therapeutic range) for a period of at least six weeks who have persistent and clinically significant positive symptoms).

57. C: Clozapine has a unique side effect profile including a rare but life-threatening side effect of agranulocytosis. The United States FDA requires that prior to the initiation of clozapine, patients must have an absolute neutrophil count of 1500 cells/microliter or greater. An exception is made for patients diagnosed with benign ethnic neutropenia. The United States FDA also requires that patients taking clozapine have regular monitoring of neutrophil counts as well as required registry reporting.

58. D: The FDA Clozapine Risk Evaluation and Mitigation Strategy (REMS) Program requires that all patients receiving clozapine be entered into the REMS program registry and undergo regular monitoring of the absolute neutrophil count (ANC). Monitoring must occur for the duration of the therapy and is conducted weekly during the first six months of therapy followed by every other week for the second six months of therapy. After one year, monitoring should be conducted every four weeks for the entire duration of therapy.

59. B: The patient should continue the clozapine and increase the absolute neutrophil count checks to three times per week. When neutropenia develops in patients taking clozapine, interventions are based on the severity of the neutropenia. In mild neutropenia (1000-1499 cells/mcL) the recommendation is that the clozapine be continued and the frequency of monitoring increased to three times per week. In moderate neutropenia (500-999 cells/mcL) it is recommended that the clozapine be held until the absolute neutrophil count increases to 1000 cells/mcL. In severe neutropenia (<500 cells/mcL), it is recommended that clozapine be discontinued. A re-challenge is only recommended if the benefit outweighs the risk and hematology is consulted.

60. C: Clozapine-induced myocarditis is a serious side effect of clozapine treatment. In rare cases, it can rapidly progress to cardiomyopathy and heart failure. Patients on clozapine should be monitored closely for symptoms of myocarditis for at least the first four weeks of therapy. Monitoring should include vital signs, assessment for presence of symptoms, baseline EKG monitoring and weekly eosinophil count, C-reactive protein, and troponin levels. Fasting blood glucose levels may be monitored monthly during the initiation of therapy to assess for hyperglycemia. Triglyceride levels may also be monitored to assess for insulin resistance.

61. C: Psychotic symptoms can manifest as part of a primary psychiatric (psychotic) disorder or as the result of a primary medical disorder. Typical clinical presentations associated with a primary psychiatric disorder include an insidious onset, the presence of auditory hallucinations, a positive family history, onset in teens to mid-thirties and a variable presentation. Conversely, psychotic symptoms associated with a primary medical disorder are more likely to present with an acute onset, non-auditory hallucinations, onset in forties or older, family history may be variable, and presentation is often a medical or intensive care type setting.

62. C: Delusional disorder is defined as the presence of one or more delusions for a month or more in a person who does not appear odd or functionally impaired, with the exception of the delusion. There are several different subtypes of delusional disorders with persecutory and jealous subtypes occurring most commonly. In the persecutory subtype, the patient believes that he or she is being persecuted or conspired against. The grandiose subtype includes delusions that the patient has a special talent or gift or has accomplished a major achievement. The erotomanic subtype includes delusions in which the patient believes that another person is in love with him or her. In the mixed subtype, a theme does not predominate in the patient's delusions.

63. B: Hypochondriasis is defined as a preoccupation with the fear of having a serious disease despite the lack of evidence that the disease exists after appropriate medical evaluation and reassurance. Delusions of parasitosis is the most common form of monosymptomatic hypochondriacal psychosis. Other forms include delusions of dysmorphism, delusions of halitosis and delusions of body odor. In delusional parasitosis, the patient experiences the delusion that they are infected by bugs, worms, or parasites. Patients diagnosed with this rare condition are usually functional, with a small percentage experiencing a disruption in activities of daily living.

64. A: The serotonin norepinephrine reuptake inhibitors (SNRI's) all have the potential to increase blood pressure with the exception of duloxetine. Prior to initiation of an SNRI other than duloxetine, blood pressure should be assessed and then monitored throughout therapy. Appropriate anti-hypertensive therapy can be initiated in patients that are hypertensive prior to the start of therapy with an SNRI. Typically, blood pressure is initially monitored every 1-2 weeks for the first month of therapy and then every 1-2 months for the next six months of therapy. After the 6-7 months of therapy, monitoring can then be moved to every 3-6 months depending on the medication, dose, and patient response.

65. D: Serotonin norepinephrine reuptake inhibitors (SNRI's) are used in the treatment of depression. They work by blocking presynaptic serotonin and norepinephrine transporter proteins, thereby inhibiting the reuptake of these neurotransmitters. Patients receiving SNRI's should receive information on drug interactions, side effects, stopping the medication, and response time. Patients should be notified that it may take several weeks to see a full response. Side effects of SNRI's include dizziness, diaphoresis, hypertension, and sexual dysfunction. Nausea is the most common side effect, and patients should be advised to take their medication with food to minimize nausea. SNRI's should be tapered when discontinued and not abruptly discontinued.

66. A: The enzyme monoamine oxidase is distributed in tissues throughout the body. It is responsible for the oxidative deamination of serotonin, norepinephrine, and dopamine. It is made up of two components, MAO-A and MAO-B. MAO-B is responsible for the metabolization of phenylethylamine. MAO-A is responsible for the breakdown of serotonin and norepinephrine. Together MAO-A and MAO-B break down dopamine. Monoamine oxidase inhibitors work by blocking monoamine oxidase.

67. B: There are several food and beverages that should be prohibited in patients taking monoamine oxidase inhibitors. These foods and beverages often contain significant amounts of tyramine that can interact with monoamine oxidase inhibitors (MAOIs), or potentially with selective MAOI-b inhibitors at high doses. This can result in elevated blood pressure or hypertensive crisis. Foods and beverages that should be strictly avoided include draft beers, vermouth, all aged cheeses including any food items that contain aged cheeses, all aged smoked, pickled, or cured meats, fish or poultry, soy products, fava or broad beans, any over-ripened or dried fruit including avocado and bananas, and all aged or fermented soy and yeast products. There are multiple other food and beverage items in which intake should be minimal (no more than ½ cup serving of 1-3 of the food/beverage items on the list per day). These include caffeinated drinks, red or white wine, clear alcoholic spirits, sour cream, other cheeses (such as American, mozzarella, parmesan), pepperoni, bologna, hot dogs, chili peppers, raspberries, canned figs, and chocolate.

68. B: In 2006, the United States FDA approved selegiline in the form of a transdermal patch for the treatment of depression. The transdermal delivery of selegiline allows for avoidance of direct inhibition of MAO-A in the gastrointestinal tract. The recommended starting and target dose is 6 mg/day. At this dose, dietary restrictions are not required. The maximum recommended dose for transdermal selegiline is 12 mg/day. Dose increases should occur in increments of 3 mg/day at a minimum interval of at least 2 weeks.

69. B: The DSM-5-TR includes a group of somatic disorders that are characterized by the presence of prominent somatic symptoms as well as substantial distress and psychosocial impairment. This category includes somatic symptom disorder, illness anxiety disorder, functional neurological symptom disorder (conversion disorder), factitious disorder, and psychological factors affecting other medical conditions. A DSM-5-TR diagnosis of illness anxiety disorder must meet the following criteria: preoccupation with having or acquiring a serious, undiagnosed illness, mild or nonexistent somatic symptoms, substantial anxiety in regards to health including a low threshold for becoming alarmed about one's health, excessive behaviors related to health or avoidance of situations or activities that could be a potential health threat, illness preoccupation is present for at least six months and is not better explained by other mental disorders. Hypochondriasis and somatoform disorders are diagnoses listed in the DSM-IV-TR.

70. C: Conversion disorder (also known as functional neurological symptom disorder) is characterized by neurologic symptoms such as weakness, non-epileptic seizures, and abnormal movements. While these symptoms cause distress and impairment, there is no connection between the symptoms and a neurologic disease. First line treatment for patients with conversion disorder is patient education regarding the diagnosis. Cognitive behavioral therapy and physical therapy are additional treatment option. Some patients may benefit from pharmacotherapy, with the most commonly used medications being antidepressants.

71. A: For agitated patients that are intoxicated with a central nervous system depressant (including alcohol), droperidol or haloperidol IM or IV are the recommended pharmacologic treatment options. Lorazepam and Midazolam are recommended for agitated patients that are intoxicated with a central nervous system stimulant. Risperidone may be utilized in agitated patients who are cooperative.

72. C: Acute delirium and subsequent violent behavior can be caused by a multitude of both medical and psychiatric disorders/conditions. The mnemonic "FIND ME" can assist clinicians in determining the etiology of acute delirium and violence. F stands for functional causes (for example psychiatric), I stands for infectious, N stands for neurologic, D stands for drugs, M stands for metabolic and E stands for endocrine.

73. D: "Spice gold" is an example of a synthetic cannabinoid, a chemically synthesized analog of natural cannabinoids. Synthetic cannabinoids are recreational drugs commonly used in younger males age 20-30. The clinical effects are similar to natural marijuana intoxication; however, their use may result in more severe life-threatening symptoms due to the addition of other chemical analogs. Synthetic cannabinoid use can result in hyperthermia and rhabdomyolysis in cases of severe intoxication. Rhabdomyolysis is characterized by myalgias, generalized weakness, reddish brown urine, and a markedly elevated serum creatinine kinase level. Hyperthermia, muscle rigidity, seizures, and agitation can lead to rhabdomyolysis. If not promptly treated, rhabdomyolysis can quickly result in acute renal failure. Hyperkalemia commonly occurs in patients with rhabdomyolysis, secondary to massive muscle breakdown.

74. B: Administration of 2 mg of lorazepam IV may be considered for a cathinone overdose. Patients intoxicated with synthetic cathinones (also known as bath salts) typically present with tachycardia, hypertension, hyperthermia, diaphoresis, agitation, anxiety, and violent behavior. Chest pain and heart palpitations may also accompany hypertension and tachycardia. First line treatment for agitation associated with cathinone overdose is intravenous administration of a benzodiazepine. Haloperidol is not recommended as first line treatment in cathinone overdose due to its potential to prolong the QTc interval and lower seizure threshold. Hypertension is generally managed by the use of intravenous benzodiazepines. Refractory hypertension may be treated using intravenous anti-hypertensives such as nitroprusside. Gastric lavage is not recommended unless large doses of amphetamines have been ingested orally or the patient presents for medical care within one hour of the ingestion.

75. C: Anticholinergic poisoning is characterized by cutaneous vasodilation (red as a beet), anhidrosis (dry as a bone), anhidrotic hyperthermia (hot as a hare), nonreactive mydriasis, mental status changes (mad as a hatter) including agitation, anxiety, confusion, disorientation, delirium, psychosis, coma and seizures, and urinary retention (full as a flask). Other symptoms may include tachycardia and decreased or absent bowel sounds. Sympathomimetic overdose and serotonin toxicity may also cause agitation, hyperthermia, and tachycardia but can usually be distinguished from anticholinergic poisoning. Hyperpnea is a classic symptom of salicylate poisoning as salicylates stimulate the medullary respiratory center causing tachypnea and hyperventilation.

76. B: Mirtazapine is the least likely to interact with other medications. The atypical antidepressant agomelatine is contraindicated in patients taking medications that potently inhibit the enzyme CYP1A2, the enzyme that works to metabolize agomelatine in the liver. The atypical antidepressant bupropion is metabolized in the liver by the P450 hepatic cytochrome enzyme 2B6. Patients taking bupropion should avoid taking medications that inhibit this enzyme as it may increase the plasma concentration of bupropion, thereby increasing the risk of seizures. Maprotiline is not an atypical antidepressant and has the potential for multiple drug interactions. Drug-drug interactions are less problematic with mirtazapine as mirtazapine is not a potent or moderate inhibitor of hepatic cytochrome P450 enzymes.

77. C: Bupropion is an atypical antidepressant that is used in the treatment of major depression, seasonal affective disorder, attention deficit hyperactivity disorder, obesity, tobacco dependence, and hypoactive sexual disorder. Contraindications in the use of bupropion include bulimia nervosa, anorexia nervosa, seizure disorders, the use of monoamine oxidase inhibitors within the past 2 weeks, and abrupt withdrawal from alcohol, benzodiazepines, or other sedatives. Caution should also be utilized in patients who are concurrently taking medications that lower seizure threshold.

78. C: Triggering events are common and may include acute emotional events and physical events as well as chronic emotional stress. Transient global amnesia (TGA) is characterized by a reversible anterograde amnesia accompanied by repetitive questioning. It commonly occurs in middle-aged and elderly patients. Episodes of transient global amnesia are distinct with a well-defined time of onset. The mean duration of episodes is six hours. A past history of a similar episode is rare. Triggering events are common and may include acute emotional events, physical events, medical procedures, changes in altitude, changes in body temperature, or chronic emotional stress. Symptoms that may accompany the episode include headache, nausea, paresthesias, and dizziness.

79. B: There are many proposed theories on the pathophysiology of transient global amnesia. A psychogenic origin was originally postulated when the disorder was first recognized, however it is theorized that transient global amnesia is an organic disorder with psychogenic stressors playing a contributing role. Migraines, venous congestion, and arterial insufficiency are all proposed theories on the etiology of transient global amnesia; however, the pathogenesis remains unknown. The primary site of the neurologic disturbance is the medial temporal lobe.

80. C: There are many second-generation antipsychotics that cause prolongation of the QT interval, thereby increasing the risk of torsades de pointes and lethal arrhythmias. Iloperidone and ziprasidone carry a slightly higher risk for QT prolongation than other second-generation antipsychotics. Quetiapine is also associated with QT prolongation and carries a cautionary statement for use in patients with cardiac risk. Olanzapine is associated with mild QT prolongation. Aripiprazole, lurasidone, brexpiprazole, and cariprazine are the least likely second-generation antipsychotics to cause cardiac arrhythmias.

81. A: Neuroprotective therapy in the treatment of Parkinson's disease is still theoretical with some neuroprotective pharmacologic agents showing promise in the treatment of animals and/or humans. With the lack of current evidence to support these agents as a proven treatment option to slow the progression of Parkinson's, a great majority of the pharmacologic agents utilized are designed to treat symptoms. The pharmacologic agents that have shown promise in the treatment option of Parkinson's disease are selegiline and rasagiline (both monoamine oxidase inhibitors) and coenzyme Q10. Vitamin E has not shown effectiveness as a neuroprotective agent in the treatment of Parkinson's disease.

82. C: Communication is not one of the six principles of trauma informed care. The Substance Abuse and Mental Health Services Administration (SAMHSA) has six guiding principles that comprise a trauma informed approach and trauma specific interventions to address the consequences of trauma and promote healing. The six principles include safety, trustworthiness and transparency, peer support, collaboration and mutuality, empowerment, choice and voice, and cultural, historical and gender issues. According to SAMHSA, a trauma informed program should realize the impact of trauma and have an understanding of the paths to recovery; recognize the signs and symptoms of trauma; respond by integrating knowledge of trauma into policies, procedures, and clinical practice; and seek to actively resist re-traumatization.

83. A: DSM-5-TR diagnosis of psychological factors affecting other medical conditions (PFAOMC) includes the following criteria: a general medical symptom or disorder is present, psychological or behavioral factors have a negative impact on the medical condition by posing additional health risks to the patient, psychological or behavioral factors aggravate the underlying pathophysiology or exacerbate symptoms, and/or psychological or behavioral factors disrupt the treatment of the general medical condition. In addition, other mental disorders do not explain the psychological or behavioral factors.

84. D: Adjustment disorder is characterized by the development of psychological distress or behavioral symptoms as a result of a general medical disorder. When psychological distress or behavioral symptoms exacerbate symptoms of a general medical disorder, a diagnosis of psychological factors affecting other medical conditions (PFAOMC) is made. In some instances, a

44

patient's emotional state aggravates and is aggravated by the medical disorder. In this case, both adjustment disorder and psychological factors affecting other medical conditions are diagnosed. A DSM-5-TR diagnosis of illness anxiety disorder must meet the following criteria: preoccupation with having or acquiring a serious, undiagnosed illness, mild or nonexistent somatic symptoms, substantial anxiety in regard to health including a low threshold for becoming alarmed about one's health, excessive behaviors related to health or avoidance of situations or activities that could be a potential health threat, illness preoccupation is present for at least six months and is not better explained by other mental disorders.

85. A: Non-emancipated minors have a patient representative (usually a parent or guardian) that has the right to make health care decisions for them and access their medical records. Under the Health Insurance Portability and Accountability Act, an adolescent is considered an individual (enabling them to obtain access to their medical records, obtain copies and request corrections, and authorize the disclosure of private health information) when the minor has the right to consent to health care and does consent, when the minor may legally receive care without parental consent and the minor or a third party (i.e. court) can consent to the care, and when a parent is in agreement with a statement of confidentiality between the healthcare provider and the minor patient and this is formally documented in the medical record.

86. D: The Family Educational Rights and Privacy Act (FERPA) allows parents access to their minor's educational records. If these records contain any health information, that information is also accessible by the parents. In the event that health records are housed separately in a school-based health center, parental access would not be covered by FERPA. HIPAA law would apply in this circumstance and parental access would be dependent on state law, the minor's ability to provide consent and the confidentiality of information within the medical record. The Confidentiality of Medical Information Act (CMIA) is a medical privacy law specific to the state of California. The Children's Online Privacy Protection Rule (COPPA) requires operators of websites or online services for children to meet certain requirements.

87. B: Parents are not financially liable for emancipated unless they have agreed to pay for the service, the parent is involved in the treatment plan, or the minor lives at home and the treatment is deemed necessary. Emancipated minors are also typically financially responsible for the healthcare services that they receive regardless of whether or not the treatment is emergent. Confidentiality can be breached when a bill for healthcare services for an adolescent patient is sent to a parent or guardian for payment. Some clinics may opt to not bill for certain services to avoid the risk of a breach in confidentiality.

88. A: A conscience clause is defined as a provision in the legislation that allows a pharmacist, physician, or other health care provider not to provide certain medical services for religious reasons or conscience. This provision is often associated with issues related to abortion, sterilization, and contraception; however, it may include other aspects of patient care. Several states have legislation that includes specific conscience clauses.

89. B: Problems with concentration is considered an arousal symptom in acute stress disorder. The presence of at least nine symptoms from the categories of intrusion, negative mood, dissociation, avoidance, and arousal, beginning or worsening after the traumatic event occurred are part of the diagnostic criteria for acute stress disorder according to the DSM-5-TR. Recurrent, involuntary, and intrusive distressing memories of the traumatic event and dissociative reactions are classified as intrusive symptoms. The persistent inability to experience positive emotions is classified as a negative mood symptom. Problems with concentration are included in the arousal symptoms along with hypervigilance, sleep disturbance, irritable behavior, problems with concentration, and an exaggerated startle response.

90. D: The recommended initial approach to patients on a selective serotonin reuptake inhibitor (SSRI) that experience sexual dysfunction is to wait for spontaneous remission of sexual impairment. The estimated incidence of sexual dysfunction related to selective serotonin reuptake inhibitors is 50%. A phosphodiesterase-5 inhibitor may be utilized for female patients with sexual dysfunction, however adding on bupropion at a higher dose is recommended over the use of a phosphodiesterase-5 inhibitor. The recommended treatment option for patients on an SSRI who experience severe sexual dysfunction but are significantly benefiting from SSRI therapy is switching antidepressants as opposed to augmenting the SSRI with a second medication.

91. C: The therapeutic technique of simple reflection can be used to help build empathy. Examples of simple reflection include reflection on affect (for example "You seem upset") or reflection content (for example "Sounds as if your sister is a big support to you."). Clarification, normalizing, and giving recognition are therapeutic communication techniques that can be beneficial in gentle inquiry and instilling hope.

92. B: "Many people tell me that when they are feeling very depressed, they sleep a lot more than usual. Has this ever happened to you?" The therapeutic technique of normalizing can be used in the process of gentle inquiry or for exploration and clarification of an issue or problem. Normalizing situations can be helpful in gathering more information about a problem or issue and may help the client to feel that they are not the only one with the problem or behavior. Using broad openings ("What brings you in to see me today?"), giving recognition or positive affirmation ("You are concerned about being a good wife."), and simple clarification ("Tell me how your depression affects you on a daily basis.") are other strategies that can be utilized in the gentle inquiry process.

93. D: A referred gate is the return to a new area of discussion by referring back to a previous statement made by the client. A natural gate involves the clinician using cues from the client's statements to bridge to new content. An implied gate joins similar regions and can provide expansion of information. Phantom gates occur when the clinician asks a question out of context, interrupting the flow of information. This technique should not be used frequently but may be necessary when more information is needed and time is a constraint.

94. B: An implied gate involves the clinician moving into a new region that is topically similar to the previous region. A natural gate involves the clinician using cues from the client's previous one or two statements as well as a transitional question to bridge to a new region. A spontaneous gate occurs when the client spontaneously moves into a new region. A referred gate occurs when the clinician enters a new region by referring back to a previous statement made by the client.

95. B: Suicide attempts are made by 20-50% of patients with schizophrenia. Suicide is the leading cause of premature death amongst patients with schizophrenia. Compared to the general population, schizophrenics have an 8.5-fold greater risk of suicide. Suicide attempts are made by 20-50% of schizophrenic patients. The majority of suicides for schizophrenics occur within the first ten years of diagnosis, with 50% occurring within the first 2 years.

96. B: According to Richard Berry, MD (2012), sleep efficiency is the ratio of total sleep time to time in the bed. Non sleep related activities should not be counted in the time in the bed number. Berry defined total sleep time as the total minutes of NREM 1,2,3 and REM stages. Rapid eye movement is defined as the sleep stage characterized by fast frequency, low voltage mixed EEG, rapid eye movements and muscle atonia. Wake from sleep onset during time in bed to lights on is defined as wake after sleep onset.

97. D: Sleep onset insomnia is defined as the inability to fall asleep during typical sleeping times (point of normal sleep onset). Sleep onset insomnia may be temporary, acute, or chronic. Treatment options for sleep onset insomnia include cognitive behavioral therapy and pharmacologic agents such as ramelteon and zaleplon. Zolpidem, eszopiclone, and temazepam may be useful in the treatment of sleep maintenance insomnia. Modafinil may be useful for the treatment of hypersomnias.

98. D: Narcolepsy is defined as the brain's inability to normally regulate sleep-wake cycles. Narcolepsy is characterized by abrupt loss of muscle tone, cataplexy (strong emotional stimulation), sleep paralysis during sleep transitions, and hallucinations at the onset or end of sleep. Loud snoring, mood disturbances, fatigue, morning headache, and daytime sleepiness are symptoms that may indicate a sleep disorder. Loud snoring may also be associated with obstructive sleep apnea.

99. B: Cortisol is associated with arousal. Neurotransmitters such as serotonin, norepinephrine, dopamine, and acetylcholine stimulate arousal and wakefulness. Hormones such as cortisol and melatonin further influence arousal. Melatonin levels increase during the day in response to sunlight exposure, peak near onset of sleep, and reach a nadir near the onset of waking. Melatonin helps to promote sleep initiation and maintenance. Cortisol is associated with arousal and is inhibited by sleep. Cortisol levels increase during wake time.

100. D: Patients with obstructive sleep apnea commonly experience symptoms such as irritability, mood swings, memory or learning problems, morning headaches and depression. In obese patients, adjunct therapy may include weight loss and/or bariatric surgery. Patients with OSA should be advised to avoid alcohol or sedatives prior to bedtime. Positional therapy may also be helpful with the supine position not recommended. Patients with OSA should alert their healthcare providers especially prior to surgery as OSA may increase the risks associated with anesthesia and administration of narcotics.

101. C: Amoxapine differs from other tricyclic anti-depressants in that it is a potent norepinephrine reuptake inhibitor and it blocks postsynaptic dopamine receptors, thereby possessing antipsychotic properties. It is the only anti-depressant with anti-psychotic properties. Doxepin is a tertiary amine that more potently blocks the reuptake of serotonin in comparison with norepinephrine. Nortriptyline is a secondary amine that more potently blocks the reuptake of norepinephrine. Maprotiline is a tetracyclic antidepressant similar in structure to secondary amines, thereby more potently blocking the reuptake of norepinephrine.

102. D: Protriptyline is considered to be the "most potent" of the cyclic antidepressants. Protriptyline blocks the reuptake of both serotonin and norepinephrine, more potently blocking the reuptake of norepinephrine. The target dose of protriptyline is 15 mg-60 mg taken at bedtime. Elderly patients and patients sensitive to side effects may be started at a dose of 5 mg taken at bedtime.

103. A: Amongst the cyclic antidepressants, doxepin has the highest affinity for H1 histamine receptors, thereby increasing its sedative effect. Doxepin is also associated with a higher incidence of weight gain. The target dosing for doxepin is 150-300 mg daily, with a recommended starting dose of 25 mg at bedtime and increasing the dose by 25-50 mg every 3-4 days as side effects allow. Low dose doxepin may also be utilized for sleep maintenance insomnia.

104. C: Most cases of isolated benzodiazepine ingestion are able to be managed successfully with supportive care alone. In cases of isolated benzodiazepine overdose, a history and physical examination and regular monitoring are likely to be all that is necessary. Physical assessment should include a focus on signs of respiratory dysfunction, trauma and additional signs and symptoms present from the ingestion of co-ingestants. The observation period largely depends upon the clinical findings. Oral benzodiazepines taken without a co-ingestant rarely cause significant toxicity. Gastrointestinal decontamination with activated charcoal is not recommended as a treatment option in benzodiazepine overdose as it has not proven to be beneficial, and it increases the risk of aspiration. The use of flumazenil in the treatment of benzodiazepine overdose is controversial (may precipitate withdrawal seizures in benzodiazepine dependent patients), and it is recommended that if flumazenil is considered that consultation with a toxicologist or poison control professional occur prior to use.

105. A: Propylene glycol is the diluent used in parenteral preparations of diazepam and lorazepam. Although propylene glycol poisoning is rare, it should be considered in patients receiving large or continuous infusions of parenteral benzodiazepines (lorazepam and diazepam-propylene glycol is not the diluent for midazolam). Propylene glycol toxicity is characterized by hyperosmolarity and an anion gap metabolic acidosis. This can lead to an acute kidney injury and when severe, progress to multisystem organ failure. Treatment consists of discontinuation of the benzodiazepine and dialysis in severe cases.

106. C: Administration of diazepam would be most appropriate. Gamma hydroxybutyrate (GHB) is a drug often used in body building, the treatment of insomnia, anxiety, and alcohol dependence. It is commonly abused for its euphoric, sedative, stimulant, and sexual effects. Patients presenting with mild to moderate symptoms of gamma hydroxybutyrate (GHB) withdrawal without delirium are commonly treated with sedative-hypnotic agents to control symptoms and prevent acute decompensation. Diazepam is a recommended medication in the treatment of GHB withdrawal. Inpatient detoxification is recommended for patients with GHB withdrawal. Beta blockers are not recommended to control hypertension (caused by central sympathetic stimulation) in GHB withdrawal, rather sedatives such as diazepam are recommended to control the stimulation. Haloperidol is not recommended for the treatment of GHB withdrawal.

107. C: Gamma hydroxybutyrate (GHB) is a drug often used in body building, the treatment of insomnia, anxiety, and alcohol dependence. It is commonly abused for its euphoric, sedative, stimulant, and sexual effects. Patients presenting with gamma hydroxybutyrate (GHB) intoxication without co-intoxicants often experience hypotension, hypothermia, bradycardia, respiratory depression, agitation, amnesia, myoclonus, and seizure-like effects. Other central nervous system effects such as ataxia, nystagmus, and loss of muscle control have also been reported.

108. D: The APNA position statement on electroconvulsive therapy (2011) states that ECT is a proven therapy and further clinical trials are not needed to establish its safety and efficacy. APNA believes that ECT operated by properly trained professionals and in circumstances of medical necessity offers severely depressed patients an option that would otherwise be unavailable. The position statement goes on to say that the most significant concern about ECT treatment is treatment-related cognitive impairment, however even this symptom has been markedly lessened with all of the advances in the administration of ECT treatment. In this position statement, APNA expressed a willingness to develop standards of practice in the proper application of ECT treatment.

109. B: According to the Centers for Medicare and Medicaid Services Conditions of Participation and Interpretive Guidelines, a psychiatric advance directive is comparable to a traditional health care advance directive and should be accorded the same respect and consideration that traditional health care advance directives are given. A psychiatric advance directive may provide the patient's instructions for hospitalization, types of therapies, alternatives to hospitalization, the use of medications, and the patient's wishes regarding restraint and seclusion. It may also include naming of another person authorized to make decisions for an individual if deemed legally incompetent to make his or her own decisions. State laws vary on the use of psychiatric advance directives.

110. C: An incidental use of disclosure is defined by the Centers for Medicare and Medicaid Services (CMS) as a "secondary use or disclosure of patient information that cannot reasonably be prevented, is limited in nature, and occurs as a result of another use or disclosure that is permitted. An incidental use or disclosure is not permitted if it is a by-product of an underlying use or disclosure that violates the HIPAA privacy rule.

111. D: An incidental use of disclosure is defined by the Centers for Medicare and Medicaid Services (CMS) as a "secondary use or disclosure of patient information that cannot reasonably be prevented, is limited in nature, and occurs as a result of another use or disclosure that is permitted. An incidental use or disclosure is not permitted if it is a by-product of an underlying use or disclosure that violates the HIPAA privacy rule. An example of an incidental disclosure would be a patient visitor overhearing a registered nurse giving report on one of her patients to another registered nurse. The hospital would be expected to put reasonable safeguards in place such as training healthcare providers to speak quietly when discussing a patient's condition. A hospital is not required to eliminate all risk of incidental use or disclosure secondary to a permitted use or disclosure as long as reasonable safeguards are put into place. The other examples are all considered to be breaches according to the Health Insurance Portability and Accountability Act.

112. D: Overall, patients should be able to obtain a copy of their medical records. In limited circumstances, information may be withheld. Those circumstances include but are not limited to: psychotherapy notes, a licensed health care professional has determined that the access requested would likely endanger the life or physical safety of the individual or other person, the information contains data obtained under a promise of confidentiality (from someone other than a health care provider) and inspection could reasonably reveal the source, and a correctional institution or health care provider acting at the direction of a correctional institution may deny an inmate's request for access if access would jeopardize the health or security of the individual, other inmates, or officers or employees of the correctional facility.

113. D: A patient grievance is defined as a formal or informal written or verbal complaint regarding the patient's care that is not resolved at the time of the complaint by staff present. Grievances may also include complaints related to abuse or neglect, issues related to the hospital's compliance with the CMS Conditions of Participation, or a Medicare beneficiary billing complaint related to rights or limitations. Other complaints related to billing issues are typically not considered grievances. Information obtained from patient satisfaction surveys is not typically considered a grievance unless the patient attaches a written complaint to the survey.

114. B: The DSM-5-TR has 10 personality disorders that are grouped into three clusters based on similar characteristics. Cluster A includes paranoid, schizoid, and schizotypal personality disorders. In cluster A disorders, individuals may appear eccentric and odd. Cluster B includes histrionic, borderline, narcissistic, and anti-social personality disorders. In cluster B disorders, individuals may be erratic in their emotions or appear more dramatic and emotional in their emotions and behavior. Cluster C includes obsessive compulsive, avoidant, and dependent personality disorders. In cluster C disorders, individuals may be anxious and fearful.

115. C: The DSM-5-TR has 10 personality disorders that are grouped into three clusters based on similar characteristics. Cluster A includes paranoid, schizoid, and schizotypal personality disorders. In cluster A disorders, individuals may appear eccentric and odd. Cluster B includes histrionic, borderline, narcissistic, and anti-social personality disorders. In cluster B disorders, individuals may be erratic in their emotions or appear more dramatic and emotional in their emotions and behavior. Cluster C includes obsessive compulsive, avoidant, and dependent personality disorders. In cluster C disorders, individuals may be anxious and fearful.

116. B: Histrionic personality disorder as defined in the DSM-5-TR is a pervasive pattern of excessive emotionality and attention seeking, beginning in early adulthood and present in a variety of contexts as indicated by five or more defined characteristics. These characteristics include: feeling uncomfortable in situations in which he or she is not the center of attention, interactions with others are often characterized by inappropriate sexually seductive or provocative behavior, displays rapidly shifting and shallow expression of emotions, consistently uses physical appearance to draw attention to self, has a style of speech that is excessively impressionistic and lacking in detail, shows self-dramatization, theatricality, and exaggerated expression of emotion, is suggestible, and considers relationships to be more intimate than they actually are. The belief that he or she is special and unique and can only be understood by, or should associate with, other special or high-status people is a diagnostic criterion for narcissistic personality disorder.

117. D: Avoidant personality disorder is defined in the DSM-5-TR as a pervasive pattern of social inhibition, feelings of inadequacy, and hypersensitivity to negative evaluation, beginning by early adulthood and present in a variety of contexts. For a diagnosis of avoidant personality disorder, the presence of four (or more) defined criteria is required. Those criteria include: avoids occupational activities that involve significant interpersonal contact due to fears of criticism, disapproval, or rejection, an unwillingness to get involved with people unless certain of being liked, showing restraint within intimate relationships due to the fear of being shamed or ridiculed, being preoccupied with being criticized or rejected in social situations, being inhibited in new interpersonal situations due to the feelings of inadequacy, viewing one's self as socially inept, personally unappealing, or inferior to others, and being unusually reluctant to take personal risks or to engage in any new activities because they may prove embarrassing.

118. C: Antisocial personality disorder often begins in childhood or early adolescence and is characterized by a pattern of exploitative and socially irresponsible behaviors in which the individual does not experience guilt. Individuals with antisocial personality disorder often experience difficulty with obtaining employment and establishing stable relationships. They often fail to conform to the law and often engage in criminality. Medications are not routinely recommended in the treatment of antisocial personality disorder, as none have been proven effective. Psychodynamic and psychoanalytic therapies have not been studied in the treatment of antisocial personality disorder. Cognitive behavioral therapy is recommended for patients with mild antisocial personality disorder that possess the insight and reason to improve.

119. B: Cognitive behavioral therapy (CBT) is an effective treatment for binge eating disorder and is indicated when the patient expresses a willingness to engage in the therapy process and possesses the motivation to begin the process. Appropriate treatment goals for binge eating disorder include a reduction in binge eating episodes, a reduction in co-morbid symptoms such as anxiety and depression, and a reduction in concerns with body image. Weight loss for overweight or obese patients is not an appropriate goal as cognitive behavioral therapy is an ineffective tool for weight loss in patients with binge eating disorder.

120. C: A course of treatment using cognitive behavioral therapy in patients with binge eating disorder typically includes 20 sessions. Cognitive behavioral therapy is indicated for patients with binge eating disorder that have the desire to reduce the frequency of binge eating episodes, improve their body image and address other psychiatric co-morbidities. Cognitive behavioral therapy is not indicated for weight loss in patients with binge eating disorder. Cognitive behavioral therapy may be provided by the clinician to an individual or a group. A course of treatment usually consists of twenty sessions with a duration of 50 minutes. Therapy typically continues over a four- to five-month period and ends after the planned number of sessions are completed. Treatment may continue however if the patient's symptoms continue to significantly impede their ability to function.

121. C: Psychogenic non-epileptic seizures are not associated with a physiological dysfunction of the central nervous system. Rather, they are psychogenically determined and can mimic epileptic seizures. Psychogenic non-epileptic seizures are characterized by sudden, time-limited episodes of sensory, autonomic, cognitive, or motor disturbances. Psychogenic non-epileptic seizures are often difficult to diagnose. They are more common in females and often present in the third decade of life (although they can occur at any age). They often occur frequently and tend not to occur during sleep. They also occur more frequently in front of witnesses.

122. A: In Lewy body dementia and Parkinson's disease, visual hallucinations are characteristically complex. Visual hallucinations commonly occur in patients with Lewy body dementia and Parkinson's disease. Visual hallucinations are characteristically complex, binocular, and often occur throughout the entire visual field. In Parkinson's disease, visual hallucinations are more prevalent late in the disease course. In Lewy body dementia, visual hallucinations occur in approximately two-thirds of patients and occur earlier in the disease course. Visual hallucinations are uncommon in Alzheimer's disease.

123. D: According to the Centers for Medicare and Medicaid Services (CMS), a restraint is defined as "any manual method, physical or mechanical device, material or equipment that immobilizes or reduces the ability of a patient to move his or her arms, legs, body or head freely." The CMS definition of restraints applies to all uses of restraints in all hospital care settings. There are several common hospital practices that could meet this definition including positioning a patient's bed sheets so tightly that the patient cannot move, using side rails to prevent a patient from voluntarily getting out of bed or the use of a "freedom" splint to immobilize a patient's limb. If the patient can easily remove the device, the device would not be considered a restraint. For example, the use of a geriatric chair if the patient can remove any type of restraint appliance associated with the chair and get out of the chair on his or her own.

124. C: A patient with dementia who is experiencing agitation and anxiety is administered a high dose of a benzodiazepine to sedate the patient and keep them in bed. Medications that are utilized as a restriction to manage a patient's behavior or restrict a patient's freedom of movement and is not a standard treatment or dosage for a patient's condition is considered by the Centers for Medicare and Medicaid to be a restraint. Criteria used to determine whether the use of a drug or medication is a standard treatment or dosage for a patient's condition includes the drug being used within the pharmaceutical parameters approved by the FDA and the manufacturer for the indications that it is manufactured to address (including dosage parameters), the drug being used in adherence with national practice standards established or recognized by the medical community or professional medical associations and the drug being used to treat a specific clinical condition based on symptoms, overall clinical situation and on the knowledge of the practitioner of the patient's expected and actual response to the medication. In the example of the patient with dementia experiencing agitation, the patient has no medical symptoms that indicate a need for sedation. In this case, sedation is being used as a restraint in an attempt to keep the patient in bed.

125. A: Ketamine can exacerbate schizophrenia and should be avoided in this patient population. Ketamine is a dissociative anesthetic agent that can be useful in the treatment of acutely agitated and violent patients in which initial treatment with benzodiazepines or antipsychotics have failed and in patients with excited delirium. Clinicians may choose to avoid the use of ketamine in older patients or those with known heart disease. The recommended initial dose of ketamine for acute agitation is 1-2 mg/kg IV or 4-5 mg/kg IM. Notable side effects may include hypertension and tachycardia. In using ketamine, clinicians must be prepared to manage airway obstruction even though respiratory complications are rare. Ketamine can exacerbate schizophrenia and should be avoided in this patient population.

126. D: All of the strategies mentioned should be included. Every hospital should have a plan that outlines what to do in cases of extreme violence. Physical assault may occur even when appropriate interventions and precautions are taken. If assaulted, one should immediately summon for help. Some organizations have panic buttons which are optimal devices for staff to utilize to call for help. Maintaining a sideward posture is recommended as well as keeping the arms ready to protect one's self. If bitten, it is recommended to not pull away but rather push towards the mouth and hold the nares shut. This will increase the likelihood that the offender will open their mouth. Sudden movements should be avoided if threatened with a weapon as well as adopting a non-threatening posture. It is not recommended to reach for the weapon, even if the weapon is put down.

127. B: The Hospital Based Inpatient Psychiatric Services (HBIPS) core measure set is a quality measure set that is required for all free-standing psychiatric hospitals that are Joint Commission accredited and surveyed under the Joint Commission Comprehensive Accreditation Manual for hospitals. In addition, all inpatient psychiatric facilities reimbursed under the Inpatient Psychiatric Facility Prospective Payment System must report the six Hospital Based Inpatient Psychiatric Services (HBIPS) measures. This measure set includes the hours of physical restraint use, hours of seclusion use, patients discharged on multiple antipsychotic medications with appropriate justification, and the completion of an admission screening for violence risk, substance use, psychological trauma history and patient strengths. Alcohol use screening is part of the national hospital inpatient quality measure set on Substance Use.

128. A: The Hospital Based Inpatient Psychiatric Services (HBIPS) core measure set is a quality measure set that is required for all free-standing psychiatric hospitals that are Joint Commission accredited and surveyed under the Joint Commission Comprehensive Accreditation Manual for hospitals. In addition, all inpatient psychiatric facilities reimbursed under the Inpatient Psychiatric Facility Prospective Payment System must report the six Hospital Based Inpatient Psychiatric Services (HBIPS) measures. The numerator for the HBIPS-1 core measure is defined as patients admitted to a hospital-based inpatient psychiatric setting who are screened within the first three days of admission for all of the following: risk of violence to self or others, substance use, psychological trauma history and patient strengths. The denominator for the HBIPS-1 core measure is defined as all psychiatric inpatient discharges.

129. C: A "just culture" is one in which an atmosphere of trust encourages and rewards staff for providing safety-related information. It includes the creation of a learning culture, the design of safe systems and the management of behavioral choices. It promotes systematic improvement over individual punishment. All operational and clinical leaders including front line staff should be involved in educational sessions on just culture. Policies and procedures that authorize punishment and serve as a barrier to the implementation of a just culture should be eliminated. Policies and procedure that are based on the principles of a just culture should be adopted.

130. D: Psychological theories on anxiety include cognitive, psychodynamic, and behavioral components. Behavioral theories on anxiety focus on both classical conditioning and social learning. Neutral stimuli begin to elicit fear when frequently associated with a frightening stimulus in classical conditioning. Social learning may contribute to the development of anxiety in environments in which a child is frequently exposed to a parent's anxiety. Unresolved conflicts are associated with psychodynamic theories on anxiety.

131. D: Obsessive compulsive disorder (OCD) differs from other anxiety disorders in that numerous studies have demonstrated that the orbitofrontal cortex, anterior cingulate cortex, and striatal regions of the brain are hyperactive. This hyperactivity has been shown to lessen following treatment. In addition, a hyporeactivity of the amygdala has been noted on imaging studies of patients with OCD when exposed to nonspecific threat images.

132. A: Eye Movement Desensitization and Reprocessing (EMDR) is a type of psychotherapy that has been extensively researched and utilized in the treatment of post-traumatic stress syndrome. EMDR works by combining imaginal exposure through recalling memories of a traumatic event and cognitive restructuring. Induction of saccadic eye movements (like those seen in rapid eye movement sleep) are accomplished through the use of rhythmic finger movements by the therapist. A typical EMDR session lasts from 60-90 minutes.

133. C: Geriatric patients may express anxiety symptoms as somatic symptoms. There are multiple considerations in the treatment of the geriatric patient with anxiety. Anxiety disorders do not tend to decline with age with the exception of the patient with obsessive convulsive disorder, in which symptoms may decline with age. Generalized anxiety disorder is the most common anxiety disorder in geriatric patients. New onset panic attacks are rare in the elderly, however, if they occur, they may be attributed to medication side effects or due to other medical conditions.

134. B: A child may be diagnosed with pediatric autoimmune neuropsychiatric disorder associated with streptococcal infections (PANDAS) when obsessive compulsive disorder symptoms suddenly appear or become worse following a streptococcal infection. It is theorized that the streptococcal infection may cause inflammation of the basal ganglia causing the neuropsychiatric symptoms. PANDAS is a pediatric disorder that typically occurs from age 3 to puberty.

135. A: Patients diagnosed with pediatric autoimmune neuropsychiatric disorder associated with streptococcal infections (PANDAS) often experience additional symptoms in conjunction with their OCD. Symptoms associated with PANDAS may include hyperactivity and inattention, separation anxiety, sleep disturbances, joint pain, emotional lability, changes in muscle movements, and urinary frequency and nocturnal enuresis.

136. D: The development of postpartum psychosis is a relatively rare condition with an unknown etiology. Hormonal and genetic components are proposed factors in the development of postpartum psychosis. Postpartum psychosis is a medical emergency with the risk of suicide and infanticide being higher than that of the general population. Risk factors for the development of postpartum psychosis include a history of bipolar disorder, a history of postpartum psychosis, a family history of postpartum psychosis, the recent discontinuation of lithium or other mood stabilizing medications and first pregnancy.

137. C: Wilson's disease is a genetic disease that leads to the impairment of cellular copper transport. Neurologic manifestations of the disease are often broad, making diagnosis especially challenging. Initially, only one symptom may manifest but with disease progression a complex combination of neurologic symptoms emerges. Common neurologic symptoms include dysarthria, gait abnormalities and ataxia, drooling, Parkinsonism, dystonia, and tremor. Other symptoms such as seizures, hyperreflexia, myoclonus, urinary incontinence, and cognitive impairment may also occur.

138. B: Dysarthria is seen in the majority of patients suffering from neurologic Wilson's disease. Wilson disease is a genetic disease that leads to the impairment of cellular copper transport. The type of dysarthria varies and may include ataxic dysarthria (an irregularity in word spacing and volume) or athetoid, hypophonic or spastic speech. Parkinsonism and tremors may also be present in neurologic Wilson's disease. Parkinsonism is usually accompanied by other neurologic symptoms. Myoclonia is a less common neurologic manifestation in Wilson's disease.

139. D: Kayser-Fleischer rings are brownish or gray-green rings caused by cooper deposits in the cornea. They are typically detected by slit-lamp examination, however if sizable they may be visible without a slit-lamp examination. Kayser-Fleischer rings are seen in approximately 98% of patients with neurologic Wilson's disease and in 50% of patients with hepatic manifestations of Wilson's disease. Kayser-Fleischer rings are rarely the first clinical finding in Wilson's disease, however if Wilson's disease is suspected their presence may help in confirming the diagnosis.

140. A: Photosensitivity has been studied as a trigger for seizures with the inclusion of both natural light and artificial sources. Photic-induced seizures occur more commonly in children than adults and are usually generalized but may be focal. A propensity for photic-induced seizures may be inherited. Individuals may be sensitive to certain light triggers but not others.

141. C: Bilateral electrode placement in electroconvulsive therapy treatment involves the placement of one electrode on each temple. Bilateral placement has the greatest antidepressant efficacy as well as the fastest response time. Bilateral placement is also associated with the most memory impairment. The right unilateral electrode placement technique avoids stimulation of the left cerebral hemisphere. Right unilateral placement results in slightly lower readmission rates and causes fewer adverse cognitive effects (including memory impairment). Cognitive impairment with bifrontal electrode placement may be comparable to right unilateral electrode placement.

142. A: Leukocytosis is not a potential physiologic effect of alcohol toxicity. The toxic effects of alcohol may include irritation of the mucosa of the mouth, throat and esophagus, gastric ulceration, peripheral neuropathy (due to both alcohol related vitamin B-1 deficiency and direct contact with alcohol), thiamine deficiency, heart failure and cardiomyopathy, pancreatic tissue damage, hepatitis, and potential liver failure. Bone marrow suppression results in a decrease in red and white blood cells, as well as platelets. This places the patient at higher risk for anemia, disruptions in clotting, and infection.

143. B: Wernicke-Korsakoff syndrome is a neurological syndrome that occurs with a thiamine deficiency. Symptoms of Wernicke-Korsakoff syndrome include nystagmus, ataxia, paralysis of ocular muscles, confusion, apathy, and somnolence. The syndrome is also manifested by extreme loss of retentive memory. With thiamine supplementation over several months, symptoms may improve; however, memory loss may be permanent.

144. D: The American Society of Addiction Medicine's Patient Placement Criteria (ASAM PPC-2R) includes five levels of care in the continuum of substance abuse treatment. These levels are as follows:

- Level 0.5—Early intervention
- Level 1—Outpatient treatment
- Level 2—Intensive outpatient/partial hospitalization treatment
- Level 3—Residential/inpatient treatment
- Level 4—Medically managed intensive inpatient services

145. C: Thiamine 100 mg IM/IV daily or 100 mg P.O. three times daily for three days, followed by 100 mg P.O. daily. Thiamine is an essential component of alcohol intoxication and withdrawal as it serves as a neuroprotective agent. The typical dosing for thiamine in alcohol intoxication/withdrawal is 100 mg IM/IV daily or 100 mg P.O. three times daily for three days, followed by 100 mg P.O. daily. In addition, oral folate (1 mg) and a multivitamin are typically administered daily in conjunction with the thiamine.

146. C: Librium is utilized in the treatment of alcohol intoxication and withdrawal. It can be tapered up for worsening alcohol withdrawal symptoms or down to lessen sedation. It has a long half-life (30-100 hours) and is metabolized by the liver. Librium is only effective when administered orally, as it is poorly absorbed intramuscularly and cannot be administered intravenously. Symptoms that indicate a reduction in dose may be needed include ocular nystagmus, ataxia, and slurred speech.

147. D: Disulfiram is an alcohol-sensitizing agent that is used to deter people from drinking alcohol. It works by stopping the hepatic enzyme that breaks up acetaldehyde. The presence of acetaldehyde in the blood creates an illness which may include flushing, tachycardia, hypotension, nausea, dizziness, shortness of breath, and confusion. Disulfiram is contraindicated in patients with liver disease, those at high risk for alcohol abuse relapse, viral hepatitis carriers, and those who work in factories where fumes are inhaled.

148. B: Naltrexone is an opiate antagonist that is utilized in the treatment of both alcohol and/or opiate addiction to decrease cravings. It is available orally and in depo injection form. The depo form is administered as a monthly injection (typically injected into the gluteal muscles). Side effects include pain at the injection site, insomnia, and feelings of "depersonalization." The depo form of the naltrexone is expensive and complex in its preparation, requiring refrigeration and reconstitution.

149. C: The dosing of methadone varies widely amongst patients and differs significantly when utilized for opioid addiction as opposed to pain management. Methadone is typically administered in a single daily dose with the initial dose dependent on the time of last opioid use, amount used, and if the patient has experienced a reduction in tolerance. Most opioid treatment programs provide a first day dose of 30 mg. An additional 10 mg can be administered if the patient experiences significant withdrawal symptoms after the 30 mg dose. It is recommended that the first day dose not exceed 40 mg.

150. A: In order to be eligible for methadone maintenance in the United States, prospective patients must have documentation of the presence of an opioid use disorder for at least one year of continuous use and be at least 18 years of age or older. Exceptions to these criteria include pregnancy even when the opioid use has been less than one year, patients recently released from hospitalization or incarceration with a history of an opioid use disorder and a documented likelihood of relapse of opioid use, and physiologic dependence by a clinician. In addition, patients who have been on methadone maintenance within the past two years are exempt from demonstrating current physical dependence or a current opioid use disorder if the clinician documents a likelihood of relapse. Patients are required to attend individual counseling (as clinically indicated) however, it does not determine eligibility.

151. C: Buprenorphine is a schedule III controlled substance (in the United States) that is utilized in the long term treatment of patients with opioid dependence to reduce illicit opioid use. The use of buprenorphine is limited to those clinicians that are certified and specially trained and have registered with the United States Center for Substance Abuse Treatment (CSAT) or the Substance Abuse and Mental Health Services Administration (SAMHSA) as well as the Drug Enforcement Administration (DEA). Regulations specific to buprenorphine include the capacity to provide or refer patients for counseling when providing office-based buprenorphine, performing induction either in a clinician's office under observation or at the patient's home, and the ability of a clinician to treat a hospitalized patient without a DEA waiver.

152. C: The recommended treatment for patients with moderate to severe opioid use disorder includes maintenance treatment with medication rather than abstinence-based treatment. In patients with a mild opioid use disorder, naltrexone is the recommended choice of medications. In patients with moderate to severe opioid use disorder, buprenorphine is recommended over other medications. Methadone has a higher risk of lethal overdose in this population. Levo-alpha-acetylmethadol is no longer being manufactured due to the increased risk of cardiac arrhythmias associated with its use.

153. B: The use of methadone in therapeutic doses, as well as in overdoses, has been associated with the prolongation of the QTc interval and torsades de pointes. In many of the patients that have developed torsades de pointes when taking methadone, other risk factors for the development of an arrhythmia have been present. It is recommended that prior to the initiation of methadone, the patient be informed of the potential risk of arrhythmia and that other risk factors for QTc prolongation and patient history of structural heart disease, arrhythmia or syncope is assessed. Current evidence does not support obtaining a baseline echocardiogram prior to initiation of methadone. Potential risks and benefits of methadone therapy should be discussed with patients that have a QTc interval greater than 450 msec but less than 500 msec and ECG monitoring should occur.

154. A: According to the Centers for Medicare and Medicaid (CMS), hospitals must report the following deaths associated with restraint and seclusion directly to CMS no later than the close of business on the next business day following knowledge of the patient's death: each death that occurs while a patient is in restraint or seclusion, excluding those in which only 2-point soft wrist restraints were used and the patient was not in seclusion at the time of death, each death that occurs within 24 hours after the patient has been removed from restraint or seclusion, excluding those in which only 2-point soft wrist restraints were used and the patient was not in seclusion within 24 hours of their death, and each death known to the hospital that occurs within one week after restraint or seclusion where it is reasonable to assume that use of restraint or placement in seclusion contributed directly or indirectly to a patient's death, regardless of the type(s) of restraint used on the patient during this time. A death that occurred while a patient was in restraints but not seclusion and the only restraints used on the patient were applied exclusively to the patient's wrist(s) and were composed solely of soft, non-rigid, cloth-like materials must be recorded in an internal hospital log or other system that is immediately available to CMS upon request.

155. D: The CMS Condition of Participation (482.13 (f)(1)) related to staff competency in the use of restraints states that all staff having direct patient care responsibilities must demonstrate competency in the use of restraints prior to participating in the application of restraints; implementation of seclusion; and the monitoring, assessment, or care of a patient in restraints or seclusion. In addition, competency must be demonstrated initially as part of the orientation process as well as periodically based on what is outlined in the hospital's policy.

156. B: Lesch-Nyhan syndrome is a complex motor-behavioral condition that occurs from genetic mutations for the coding of the enzyme hypoxanthine-guanine phosphoribosyltransferase (HPRT). This results in deficient enzyme activity. It is inherited as an X-linked recessive trait. The severity of the disease is associated with the level of enzyme deficiency. Boys affected by this syndrome have developmental delays, intellectually disabled, and extrapyramidal and pyramidal motor symptoms. Self-mutilating behavior is also associated with Lesch-Nyhan syndrome.

157. C: According to the Taskforce on Childhood Movement Disorders, stereotypies are defined as "repetitive, simple movements that can be voluntarily suppressed." Movements are typically simple back and forth movements that involve the upper extremities. Lower extremities are typically not involved. Common stereotypies include repetitive chewing, rocking, tapping, twirling, or touching. Stereotypies can be stopped by distraction and typically occur in children with intellectual disabilities or developmental disorders; however, they can also occur in otherwise normal children. Rett syndrome is an example of a disorder characterized by marked stereotypies.

158. D: Sydenham chorea is a clinical manifestation of rheumatic fever and is the most common form of acquired chorea amongst children. Psychiatric symptoms include irritability, distractibility, and age-regressive behavior. Sydenham chorea is also associated with obsessive-compulsive symptoms with the disorder being diagnosed in a proportion of Sydenham chorea patients. Obsessive-compulsive symptoms can occur prior to, concurrent with, or after the onset of Sydenham chorea.

159. D: There are multiple conditions that can cause acquired chorea. Autoimmune or inflammatory disorders, metabolic and endocrine disorders, infectious diseases, toxins, and certain medications are all potential causes. Medications that have the potential to cause chorea include anticonvulsants, central nervous system stimulants, calcium channel blockers, dopamine blocking and depleting agents, antihistamines, benzodiazepines, and certain types of anti-depressants.

160. A: Tardive dyskinesia is much less common in children than adults. Tardive dyskinesia is a hyperkinetic movement disorder associated with the use of dopamine receptor blocking antipsychotic agents. The onset of tardive dyskinesia is gradual, most commonly occurring during treatment with the antipsychotic medication. It may occur as early as 1-6 months after the initiation of treatment. Tardive dyskinesia is likely to appear after a dose reduction or switching to a less potent antipsychotic medication. It may also occur following discontinuation of the drug. The hypokinetic effect of the antipsychotic medication may mask the symptoms of tardive dyskinesia. Tardive dyskinesia is often reversible and occurs more commonly in adults than children.

161. D: According to the Centers for Medicare and Medicaid, when restraint or seclusion is used to manage violent or self-destructive behavior, a face-to-face assessment of the patient must occur within one hour after the initiation of the intervention. This is also applicable when a medication is used as a restraint to manage violent or self-destructive behavior. This evaluation may be conducted by a physician or licensed independent practitioner, a registered nurse, or a physician assistant with the appropriate training to conduct the one-hour face to face evaluation as defined by CMS. The evaluation must be conducted in person.

162. C: Tardive dystonia is a subtype of tardive dyskinesia in which more sustained dystonic manifestations such as shoulder and jaw dystonia, retrocollis, opisthotonus, hyperextension of the arms and legs and blepharospasm predominate. Late-appearing motor restlessness occurs in tardive akathisia. Transient tardive dyskinesia is limited to a relatively short period of time during the course of treatment with antipsychotic drugs followed by spontaneous resolution. Tachypnea, irregular breathing rhythms and grunting noises occur in respiratory dyskinesia.

163. C: Neuroferritinopathy is a neurodegenerative disorder that results from an accumulation of iron in the brain. Iron accumulates in the basal ganglia due to a mutation in the FTL gene encoding the ferritin light chain. Symptoms associated with neuroferritinopathy include extrapyramidal features such as chorea, Parkinsonism, and dystonia. Cognitive impairment is also typically associated with neuroferritinopathy.

164. B: For patients presenting to the emergency department setting for evaluation of an acute, new-onset seizure, computed tomography is recommended due to its quick availability to alert practitioners to acute neurologic problems that require intervention. CT is relatively insensitive comparted to magnetic resonance imaging; therefore, MRI is the recommended option for patients with new-onset epilepsy to identify possible structural causes that may include brain tumor, vascular malformation, dysplasia, or hippocampal sclerosis.

165. C: Primary progressive aphasia is defined as a clinical syndrome in which language becomes impaired by deficits in word finding, word comprehension, word usage, and sentence construction. Its onset is usually insidious with a gradual progression of deficits. Primary progressive aphasia occurs when neurodegenerative disease affects the language dominant hemisphere of the brain. There are three variants of primary progressive aphasia including nonfluent, semantic, and logopenic. In the logopenic variant, patients experience an impairment of single-word retrieval and repetition with errors in speech and naming. Single word comprehension, motor speech, and object knowledge are not affected. Agrammatism is also absent in this variant.

166. D: Other psychiatric disorders may occur in conjunction with attention deficit hyperactivity disorder in adults, including mood and anxiety disorders, substance use disorder, and intermittent explosive disorder. Attention deficit hyperactivity disorder, a common disorder diagnosed in childhood and adolescence, often continues into adulthood. The predominant symptom of adult attention deficit hyperactivity disorder is inattention. Symptoms of hyperactivity and impulsivity are less overt in adults. Symptoms of inattention in adults tend to involve an inability to focus on a task, especially for long periods of time. Adult ADHD patients may struggle with organization and time management. ADHD in adults may occur in conjunction with other psychiatric disorders including mood and anxiety disorders, substance use disorder and intermittent explosive disorder.

167. B: In adult attention deficit hyperactivity disorder (ADHD), deficits in executive function are often seen. Executive function is defined as "self-directed actions needed to choose goals and create, enact and sustain actions toward those goals" Examples of executive dysfunction include deficits in working memory, self-monitoring, initiation, self-inhibition, and task-shifting. Executive dysfunction often results in difficulties with time management, organization, prioritization, and memory. Mood lability and motivational deficits are associated with emotional dysregulation that occurs in ADHD.

168. D: Assertive community treatment is defined as an integrated community-based model utilized for the delivery of clinical and social services to individuals with severe mental illness. It is indicated for patients with severe mental illness with a recent history of repeated hospitalization or homelessness. The goal of assertive community treatment is to assist patients in maintaining a community-based residence and to help them adhere to their prescribed medication regimen. An additional goal is the minimization of inpatient or emergency services.

169. B: Ketamine may be used as an anesthetic agent for electroconvulsive therapy treatment. It appears to initially enhance the benefits of ECT; however, the benefits tend to dissipate throughout the course of ECT treatment. Ketamine should be used cautiously in patients with heart disease as it may cause hypertension in higher doses. Post-disorientation can occur when ketamine is utilized in ECT treatment. Ketamine can prolong or enhance ECT seizures because it is less anticonvulsant than other anesthetic agents.

170. C: Electroconvulsive therapy is used primarily in the treatment of severe unipolar depression. It may also be indicated in the treatment of other illnesses including bipolar disorder, schizophrenia, delirium, schizoaffective disorder, and neuroleptic malignant syndrome. ECT has not shown efficacy in the treatment of milder depressions including dysthymic disorder and adjustment disorder with depressed mood. ECT may also be used to treat the motor symptoms associated with Parkinson's disease, refractory status epilepticus, and chronic pain syndromes.

171. C: The Mental Health First Aid Act of 2015 authorizes funding for mental health first aid training programs to train participants in the recognition of symptoms of mental illness and substance use disorders, the safe de-escalation of crisis situations, and the initiation of timely referrals to available community resources for those suffering from mental health and substance use disorders. The Mental Health Study Act of 1955 called for "an objective, thorough, nationwide analysis and reevaluation of the human and economic problems of mental health." The Mental Health Reform Act ensures that mental health programs are effectively serving those with mental illness and works to assist states in meeting the needs of mental health patients. The Helping Families in Mental Health Crisis Act has not yet been passed into law.

172. B: In Peplau's theory of interpersonal relations, the roles of the nurse include stranger, teacher, resource person, counselor, surrogate, and leader. The role of the nurse as a resource person is "one who provides specific needed information that aids in the understanding of a problem or new situation." The role of the nurse as a teacher is "one who imparts knowledge in reference to a need or interest." The role of the nurse as a counselor is defined by Peplau as "one who helps to understand and integrate the meaning of current life circumstances and provide guidance and encouragement to make changes." The role of the nurse as a leader is "to help the client assume maximum responsibility for meeting treatment goals in a mutually satisfying way."

173. C: According to Peplau's theory of interpersonal relations, there are four identified, sequential phases in the interpersonal relationship. In the orientation phase, direction is given by the nurse as the nurse engages the client in treatment and provides information. In the identification phase, the client works interdependently with the nurse and begins to express feelings and feel stronger. In the exploitation phase, the client makes full use of services offered. In the resolution phase, the client gives up dependent behavior and the nurse-client relationship ends.

174. B: Peplau defines four levels of anxiety in her theory of interpersonal relations including mild, moderate, severe, and panic. Peplau defines mild anxiety as "a positive state of heightened awareness and sharpened senses, allowing the person to learn new behaviors and solve problems." In mild anxiety, the client can take in all available stimuli. In moderate anxiety the client experiences a decrease in perceptual field. The client can only solve problems or learn new behavior with assistance. In severe anxiety, the client experiences feelings of dread or terror. They cannot be redirected to a task and may experience physiologic symptoms such as chest pain or diaphoresis. In panic anxiety, the client experiences the loss of rationale thought and may experience delusions or hallucinations.

175. A: Peplau's theory of interpersonal relations includes four phases of the nurse-client relationship: orientation, identification, exploitation, and resolution. The phases of the therapeutic nurse-client are highly comparable to the nursing process. A weakness of this theory is a lesser emphasis on health promotion and maintenance. Although the concepts within this theory are highly applicable to mental health patients, this theory can be utilized for any individual with the capability and will to communicate.

Practice Test #2

1. The psychiatric-mental health nurse practitioner (PMHNP) presents data showing that a new approach to patient care has better outcomes. However, members of the staff are almost all in disagreement and spend considerable time arguing that the data are in error and providing rationales for maintaining the current approach. This is an example of:
    a. Prejudice
    b. Aggression
    c. Debate
    d. Group think

2. An effective method of handling diversity in the workplace is to:
    a. Act as though everyone is alike.
    b. Develop different standards of performance for different groups.
    c. Develop internal support systems.
    d. Attempt to solve problems quickly.

3. The PMHNP works in a community in which many people are uninsured or underinsured. The impact on health care is most likely that many of these people will:
    a. Access health care but be unable to pay bills.
    b. Postpone health care until a crisis occurs.
    c. Seek alternative forms of health care, such as a free clinic.
    d. Organize to demand better health care.

4. The PMHNP is involved in a population-based nursing intervention program. Population-based interventions are aimed at:
    a. Vulnerable or underserved subgroups within the larger population
    b. All members of the population in an area
    c. Population members who lack health insurance
    d. A specified number of individuals in the population

5. An outpatient with a long history of recurrent depression has depended on his mother for his support system, but his mother has recently entered an assisted living facility and is in poor health. The PMHNP should:
    a. Provide the patient with lists of community agencies.
    b. Assure the patient that he can manage independently.
    c. Remind the patient that the nurse practitioner is part of his support system.
    d. Assist the patient to identify other support systems.

6. From the perspective of risk management, an incident that would be classified as a "serious incident" includes which of the following?
    a. A patient falls and sprains her wrist.
    b. A patient complains that staff are rude.
    c. A patient commits suicide.
    d. A patient is raped by another patient.

7. The 3 primary components of risk analysis are (1) assessment, (2) intervention, and (3):

- a. Analysis
- b. Deliverance
- c. Communication
- d. Performance

8. The PMHNP plans to replace one screening instrument with another that is available free of cost, but to determine whether the screening instruments are equivalent (checking for validity), the nurse practitioner administers both the old and the new instruments and assesses whether positive correlation exists. This type of testing is:

- a. Convergent
- b. Divergent
- c. Predictive
- d. Multi-trait, multi-method

9. Servant leadership suggests that:

- a. All staff members of the organization serve the leader.
- b. The leader serves all others in the organization.
- c. A hierarchical system of leadership is in place.
- d. Staff members are assigned specific tasks to assist the leader.

10. The Health Insurance Portability and Accountability Act (HIPAA) (1996) privacy rules allow unrestricted disclosure of patients':

- a. Past health history
- b. Past payments for health care
- c. Future plans for health care
- d. De-identified health information

11. The PMHNP is serving on an ad hoc committee to make recommendations about process improvement and plans to begin by gathering data about the prevalence of mental health disorders, treatments, and costs. The organization that best provides this information is:

- a. Agency for Healthcare Research and Quality
- b. Substance Abuse and Mental Health Services Administration
- c. Centers for Medicare and Medicaid Services
- d. National Institute of Mental Health

12. When faced with an ethical dilemma in caring for a patient, the PMHNP should:

- a. Share concerns with others, such as an ethics committee.
- b. Try to reach a conclusion independently.
- c. Discuss the matter with a trusted friend.
- d. Try to set the concerns aside.

13. The PMHNP has been asked to evaluate a confused and delusional patient with end-stage renal disease. The nursing diagnosis that the nurse practitioner enters into the care plan is:

- a. Powerlessness
- b. Ineffective coping
- c. Disturbed thought processes
- d. Hopelessness

14. A patient taking an atypical antipsychotic medication developed dystonic reactions, including eye and neck spasms. The PMHNP prescribes:

a. Amantadine
b. Diphenhydramine
c. Propranolol
d. Clonazepam

15. In a therapeutic milieu, the primary action of the PMHNP in helping patients to develop effective interpersonal skills is:

a. Role modeling
b. Explaining expectations
c. Setting boundaries
d. Providing consequences

16. When conducting examinations of patients, the PMHNP should keep in mind that the psychiatric diagnosis for which there are the most differential diagnoses is:

a. Schizophrenia
b. Conduct disorder
c. Bipolar disorder
d. Generalized anxiety disorder

17. When using the LEARN (Listen, Explain, Acknowledge, Recommend, and Negotiate) model for cross-cultural health care, an important approach to the Explain step is to:

a. Use simple language and avoid medical jargon.
b. Use drawings, videos, and test results.
c. Wait until the patient asks for an explanation.
d. Explain to family members first whenever possible.

18. When addressing a group of older adults at a senior citizens' center about mental health, the neuroprotective strategy that the PMHNP should recommend as valuable for almost all older adults is:

a. Stopping ingestion of alcohol
b. Drinking a daily glass of wine
c. Doing physical exercise
d. Increasing social interactions

19. In a research project the PMHNP is conducting, some patients are excluded from the project; so, instead of randomized subjects, the subjects are highly selected. This type of selection could produce results that have primarily:

a. Generalizability
b. Replicability
c. External validity
d. Internal validity

20. The PMHNP sees a patient with schizophrenia taking risperidone. The patient had an electrocardiogram (ECG) performed recently that the nurse practitioner is reviewing. The PMHNP knows the ECG change that should be monitored for with risperidone is:

    a. Elevated ST segment
    b. Prolonged QT segment
    c. Depression of ST segment
    d. Absent P wave

21. The PMHNP is conducting a problem-focused office visit with an established patient in order to titrate medication. The number of elements of the psychiatric exam that must be included for CMS billing purposes is:

    a. 2-4 elements
    b. 1-5 elements
    c. 1-8 elements
    d. 11 elements

22. After a fire destroys a patient's home, the patient tells the PMHNP, "I've lost everything that's important to me. I have no money to rebuild. I don't care about anything anymore because everything is hopeless." The response that has the highest priority is:

    a. "Let's talk about the things you still have."
    b. "Do you have family and friends who can help you?"
    c. "Are you thinking about killing yourself?"
    d. "What can I do to help you cope?"

23. According to Kotter's model for organizational change, the first phase involves:

    a. Establishing a sense of urgency
    b. Developing a vision for change
    c. Empowering broad-based change
    d. Generating short-term gains

24. Sources of power in an organization usually derive from (1) authority, (2) reward, (3) expertise, and (4):

    a. Luck
    b. Deceit
    c. Enthusiasm
    d. Coercion

25. The cytochrome P450 enzyme that metabolizes approximately 50% of current drugs is:

    a. CYP1A2
    b. CYP2C9
    c. CYP2D6
    d. CYP3A4

26. A patient taking a selective serotonin reuptake inhibitor (SSRI) antidepressant (sertraline) has developed sexual side effects, including anorgasmia and reduced libido. The PMHNP recognizes the initial step in resolving this problem should be to:

    a. Change to a tricyclic antidepressant.
    b. Change to a different SSRI.
    c. Decrease dosage of the SSRI.
    d. Administer an antidote, such as sildenafil or bethanechol.

27. The relationship between the total loading dose of an administered drug and the serum concentration refers to the:

    a. Absorption
    b. Distribution
    c. Clearance
    d. Metabolism

28. When disseminating evidence regarding adverse effects associated with a medication to a large number of patients and families in a widespread area, the best method is likely:

    a. Mail/email
    b. Telephone
    c. Personal visit
    d. Group meeting

29. A patient with a history of panic attacks is admitted to the emergency department with severe chest pain and shortness of breath. The PMHNP is reviewing the patient's workup that the ER physician ordered and recognizes that the cardiac enzyme test that was ordered to best rule out a myocardial infarction is:

    a. CK-MB
    b. Myoglobin
    c. Troponin I
    d. Troponin T

30. If the PMHNP wants to follow 2 groups of adolescents (one group with a parent with substance abuse and the other a control group of adolescents whose parents are not substance abusers) to determine the incidence of substance abuse in each group, the most appropriate study design is:

    a. Randomized control trial
    b. Case-control
    c. Quasi-experimental design
    d. Cohort

31. A patient is to be included in a clinical research study. The first priority under human subject protection is to:

    a. Explain the purpose of the clinical research.
    b. Ensure that the patient meets criteria for the study.
    c. Obtain informed consent.
    d. Document patient's inclusion in the study.

32. In developing evidence-based guidelines to promote compliance with a treatment regimen, the factor that should carry the most weight in developing new policies is:

    a. Best practices identified through literature review
    b. Nursing staff preferences
    c. Physician preference
    d. Cost-effectiveness

33. The nurse practitioner is engaged in research with a screening tool to predict patients with schizophrenia who will become noncompliant with treatment. The results at the end of 24 months show that out of 200 patients, 92 (46%) were noncompliant and 88 were correctly identified (96%); 108 remained compliant, but there were 27 false-positives (25%) for noncompliance among this group. The screening test has:

    a. High sensitivity and high specificity
    b. High sensitivity and low specificity
    c. Low sensitivity and low specificity
    d. Low sensitivity and high specificity

34. An example of an interaction that promotes a therapeutic alliance between the patient and the PMHNP is the:

    a. Patient and nurse share mutual experiences.
    b. Patient and nurse discuss random topics.
    c. Patient and nurse promise to maintain secrets.
    d. Patient and nurse discuss goal setting for the patient.

35. A Hispanic patient is admitted to the unit and the PMHNP is doing the admission history, but the patient speaks very little English. The nurse practitioner should:

    a. Ask the patient's 10-year old son, who is fluent in English, to translate.
    b. Use gestures and pictures to supplement questions.
    c. Arrange for a translator.
    d. Ask the patient's wife, who speaks fair English, to answer the questions for her husband.

36. The most essential protective strategy for the PMHNP to employ to reduce the risk of legal action is to:

    a. Meet or exceed the standard of care.
    b. Maintain malpractice insurance.
    c. Document all patient care promptly.
    d. Avoid serving litigious patients.

37. A patient with a history of narcotics abuse has been taking lorazepam (Ativan) for anxiety but presents with lethargy, dizziness, headache, marked alteration in consciousness, respiratory depression, and ataxia. Her friend states the patient was found 2 hours earlier with the empty prescription bottle. The PMHNP should prescribe:

    a. Gastric emptying and charcoal
    b. Charcoal, concentrated dextrose, thiamine, and naloxone
    c. Charcoal, concentrated dextrose, and flumazenil
    d. Gastric emptying, charcoal, and naloxone

38. The PMHNP notes that a patient with frontotemporal dementia has difficulty with executive functioning, suggesting damage to the:

    a. Prefrontal cortex
    b. Premotor cortex
    c. Orbitofrontal cortex
    d. Precentral cortex

39. Ensuring that a patient has given informed consent and understands his or her rights and all of the risks and benefits of a procedure or treatment supports the ethical principal of:

    a. Beneficence
    b. Nonmaleficence
    c. Justice
    d. Autonomy

40. When assessing factors that affect readiness to learn, the PMHNP recognizes the patient's cultural background and personal goals relate to:

    a. Physical factors
    b. Mental/emotional status
    c. Experience
    d. Knowledge/education

41. The PMHNP is conducting a group with patients recovering from trauma. An action or intervention that may be viewed as retraumatization is:

    a. Utilizing a confrontational approach in the group
    b. Encouraging a patient to participate in treatment plans
    c. Screening for trauma history prior to inclusion in the group
    d. Enforcing rules of conduct in the group consistently

42. In the informal negotiations that are part of collaborating and reaching consensus, when both parties make concessions in order to reach consensus but neither side is really happy with the result, this approach to negotiation is:

    a. Accommodation
    b. Avoidance
    c. Compromise
    d. Collaboration

43. According to the general adaptation syndrome (Selye) (which comprises alarm, resistance, and exhaustion), an example of reaction to stress in the resistance stage is:

    a. Levels of neurotransmitters and hormones return to normal.
    b. The hormonal system becomes activated to produce more hormones.
    c. The body becomes exhausted and unable to sustain the stress response.
    d. Chronic health problems associated with stress arise.

44. If a patient takes 8 aspirin and promptly tells family members about taking an "overdose," and the family believes that this is a suicide attempt, but the patient did not actually intend to die but rather to get attention, this act would be classified as:

   a. Suicide ideation
   b. Suicide threat
   c. Suicide attempt
   d. Suicide gesture

45. When assessing a patient's cranial MRI, the PMHNP notes that the report indicates the patient has significant atrophy of the hippocampus. Based on this finding, the nurse practitioner should expect that the patient will have the:

   a. Inability to form new long-term memories
   b. Inability to retrieve existing long-term memories
   c. Inability to form short-term memories
   d. Inability to communicate verbally

46. When evaluating literature and information to determine the level of evidence, the category that indicates that information has supporting evidence from some studies, has a good theoretical basis, and is strongly recommended for implementation is:

   a. Category IA
   b. Category IB
   c. Category II
   d. Category III

47. When communicating with a patient, the statement by the PMHNP that exemplifies therapeutic communication is:

   a. "You should try not to worry."
   b. "Don't worry. Everything will be fine."
   c. "Why are you so upset?"
   d. "I'd like to hear how you feel about that."

48. As part of the normal aging process, changes in neurotransmitters usually occur, including:

   a. Decreased serotonin
   b. Increased epinephrine
   c. Decreased glutamate
   d. Increased acetylcholine

49. When treating anxiety in an older adult (65 years or older), the type of medication that is preferred is:

   a. A short-acting benzodiazepine
   b. A long-acting benzodiazepine
   c. A tricyclic antidepressant
   d. A β-adrenergic agent

50. A patient is taking clozapine, an antipsychotic medication, and has been a chain smoker (2 or more packs per day) for many years but is enrolled in a smoking cessation program and has not smoked for the past week. If the patient is successful at quitting smoking, the patient may:

    a. Have increased adverse effects
    b. Have no effect from smoking
    c. Require a higher dosage than normal
    d. Require a lower dosage than normal

51. When evaluating outcomes data for evidence-based practice, the type of data that includes measures of mortality, longevity, and cost-effectiveness is:

    a. Clinical
    b. Psychosocial
    c. Integrative
    d. Physiological

52. A patient with a history of anxiety (treated with lorazepam during acute episodes) and alcoholism is prescribed metronidazole for bacterial vaginosis. The PMHNP should caution the patient to:

    a. Avoid taking lorazepam during treatment.
    b. Avoid any intake of alcohol.
    c. Limit alcohol to 1 serving daily.
    d. Take lorazepam during treatment.

53. Which of the following is a tool that the PMHNP can use to provide a client's self-assessment of functional health and quality-of-life issues?

    a. Patient Health Questionnaire. (PHQ)
    b. Post-Deployment Clinical Assessment Tool (PDCAT)
    c. Barthel Index
    d. Health Status Survey (SF-36)

54. When the NP interviews a patient with chronic pain from metastatic cancer and suspected suicidal ideation, the patient states, "I can't stand this pain any more. I should just shoot myself and be done with it." The best initial response is:

    a. "I understand why you feel that way. I'll ask the doctor to prescribe an antidepressant for you."
    b. "I'm sure you don't really mean that."
    c. "Let's work together to find better ways to manage your pain."
    d. "Do you have a plan to hurt yourself?"

55. A data-heavy presentation with much raw data about progress in performance improvement is most appropriate for:

    a. Administration
    b. Nursing staff
    c. Patients
    d. All groups

56. A nurse on the psychiatric unit uses another nurse's password to access an acquaintance's electronic health record (EHR) and obtain personal information about the patient. This type of data misuse is classified as:

   a. Identity theft
   b. Unauthorized access
   c. Privacy violation
   d. Security breach

57. A 66-year-old male patient with Parkinson disease has been controlled with levodopa but has developed the on-off phenomenon with fluctuating response to the levodopa. Treatment that may be indicated to reduce the breakdown of levodopa is:

   a. Doubling the dose of oral levodopa
   b. Adding entacapone (Comtan), a COMT inhibitor
   c. Stopping treatment with levodopa
   d. Adding haloperidol (Haldol)

58. Patients receiving neuroleptics should be monitored routinely with the:

   a. Mini-Mental State Exam (MMSE)
   b. Mini-Cog
   c. Trail-Making Test
   d. Abnormal Involuntary Movement Scale (AIMS)

59. The PMHNP supports a recovery-oriented approach to a treatment program for substance abusers. A prime element of a recovery-oriented approach is:

   a. Focus on a single treatment plan for all participants.
   b. Treatment must always be voluntary.
   c. Recognition that recovery is nonlinear.
   d. The program should be community centered.

60. Staff members ask the PMHNP how to deal with a 67-year-old patient with dementia who repeatedly removes his clothing and requests sexual favors. The most appropriate response is to tell the staff to:

   a. Supervise, observe, and distract the patient.
   b. Restrict the patient to his room.
   c. Provide antipsychotic medication.
   d. Reprimand the patient.

61. A patient who has been treated for depression with an MAO inhibitor is showing inadequate response and adverse effects, so the PMHNP wants the patient to begin taking an SSRI. The nurse practitioner should:

   a. Stop the MAO inhibitor and immediately start the SSRI.
   b. Stop the MAO inhibitor and wait at least 14 days to start the SSRI.
   c. Continue the MAO inhibitor and add the SSRI in increasing doses over 1 month.
   d. Stop the MAO inhibitor and wait at least 2 months to start the SSRI.

62. The PMHNP serves as team leader on the psychiatric unit but takes on the majority of difficult tasks and often fails to delegate to other team members. The most likely reason for this is that the nurse practitioner:

    a. Is highly effective
    b. Is more knowledgeable
    c. Does not trust team members
    d. Is considerate

63. The PMHNP has been instrumental in setting up an outpatient program for patients with posttraumatic stress disorder (PTSD), but enrollment in the program and continued participation after enrollment has been low. In developing strategies to improve participation, the first place to begin is to:

    a. Review patient records.
    b. Provide incentives for participation.
    c. Survey staff members.
    d. Survey participants and eligible patients.

64. A patient has been prescribed olanzapine 15 mg daily for acute manic episodes associated with bipolar I disorder. Four days after beginning treatment, he has a sudden onset of fever (39 °C [102.2 °F]), tachypnea, and tachycardia. Oxygen saturation at rest is 93%, and he exhibits muscular rigidity and some alteration in mental status. The most likely cause of these symptoms is:

    a. Neuroleptic malignant syndrome
    b. Influenza
    c. Sepsis
    d. Tardive dyskinesia

65. In attempting to integrate evidence-based practice into patient care, the PMHNP finds that nurses' belief systems and lack of familiarity with research methods are the biggest barriers to implementing change. The best solution is to:

    a. Outline disciplinary actions for those who fail to participate.
    b. Provide incentives for participation in implementation of evidence-based practice.
    c. Provide educational programs about research- and evidence-based practice.
    d. Engage only those who are supportive of evidence-based practice.

66. The primary purpose of the Patient Self-Determination Act is to:

    a. Protect privacy of personal health information.
    b. Ensure that patients give informed consent.
    c. Ensure patients have access to health records.
    d. Protect patients from unnecessary treatments.

67. A 10-year-old child is prescribed methylphenidate for attention deficit disorder. In addition to behavioral response, the PMHNP should routinely monitor:

    a. Nutritional status and sleeping patterns
    b. Complete blood cell count
    c. Skin condition
    d. Fine and gross motor skills

68. The PMHNP is observing a group of adolescent patients with a history of drug abuse in a group therapy meeting. The group leader advised the patients that the nurse practitioner would observe their progress as part of a research project and asked them to cooperate, but this threatens external validity through:

   a. Statistical conclusion validity
   b. Selection bias
   c. Construct validity
   d. Subject reactivity

69. Two team members disagree about the best way to carry out duties, resulting in ongoing conflict and refusal to work together. The first step in resolving this conflict is to:

   a. Allow both individuals to present their side of the conflict without bias.
   b. Encourage them to reach a compromise.
   c. Tell them they are violating professional standards of conduct.
   d. Make a decision about the matter.

70. Because there is only 1 psychiatric bed available but 2 patients in need of care, the PMHNP must recommend which patient to admit. The decision regarding which patient to admit should be based on the ethical principle of:

   a. Nonmaleficence
   b. Beneficence
   c. Justice
   d. Autonomy

71. The legal procedure that authorizes the PMHNP to disclose patient personal health information is a:

   a. Subpoena
   b. Subpoena duces tecum
   c. Warrant
   d. Court order

72. A 48-year-old man reports increasing episodes of impotence that are causing anxiety and depression. The patient also reports increased thirst and frequency of urination. The initial response of the PMHNP should be to order a(n):

   a. Urinalysis
   b. Complete chem-panel
   c. Electrolyte panel
   d. Venereal disease research laboratory (VDRL) test

73. A PMHNP's scope of practice is outlined by the:

   a. American Nurses Association
   b. American Nurses Credentialing Center (ANCC)
   c. Individual state's board of nursing and Nurse Practice Act
   d. American Academy of Nurse Practitioners

74. In a just culture, when an error or accident occurs, initial fault is generally considered to be with the:

   a. Individual
   b. System
   c. Administration
   d. Training

75. A 26-year-old female patient has experienced frequent injuries because of impaired pain sensation and has exhibited increasingly careless hygiene, difficulty with writing and calculations, and frequent failure to keep appointments or keep track of time. The PMHNP recognizes that these findings may indicate abnormal brain functioning in the:

   a. Parietal lobes
   b. Frontal lobes
   c. Occipital lobes
   d. Temporal lobes

76. When conducting a physical examination of a 13-year-old girl with autism spectrum disorder, the PMHNP notes that the patient's breasts and areola have been begun to enlarge, and there is sparse dark hair evident along the labia majora. The PMHNP classifies the patient as Tanner stage:

   a. II
   b. III
   c. IV
   d. V

77. A 16-year-old patient is to be discharged from a recovery program after treatment for substance abuse. Prior to discharge, the PMHNP should:

   a. Remind the patient he is responsible for staying clean.
   b. Advise the parents to monitor all of the patient's activities.
   c. Tell the patient he must break ties with all former friends.
   d. Assist the patient to anticipate and cope with pressures.

78. The PMHNP is planning a psychoeducation program for a group of patients with schizophrenia. The most important topic to cover is:

   a. Keeping appointments
   b. Avoiding substance abuse
   c. Medication compliance
   d. Avoiding stressful situations

79. When designing a performance improvement plan, the PMHNP knows the most important consideration is:

   a. Alignment with the organization's vision, mission, goals, and objectives
   b. Cost and resources needed for implementation
   c. Determination of performance measures
   d. Determination of staff preferences and potential staff support

80. According to Erikson's psychosocial theory and stages of development, a PMHNP recognizes that a 30-year-old man who remains very insecure and dependent on his parents and still lives at home has probably not successfully achieved the stage of:

a. Trust vs mistrust
b. Identity vs role confusion
c. Industry vs inferiority
d. Initiative vs guilt

81. A 17-year-old female patient with depression has been taking fluoxetine for 10 days (10 mg daily in AM for 7 days and 20 mg daily for the last 3) but tells the PMHNP that the medication is not working as she feels the depression is unchanged. The best response is for the nurse practitioner to:

a. Increase the dose to 30 mg to increase serum level.
b. Discontinue fluoxetine and prescribe a tricyclic antidepressant.
c. Advise patient to take medication at bedtime instead of in the morning.
d. Reassure the patient that response often takes 4 weeks.

82. A patient who has had multiple arrests for driving under the influence of alcohol has agreed to begin treatment with disulfiram. Patient education should include advising the patient that:

a. The patient may experience severe illness if they drink alcohol.
b. The patient should avoid driving.
c. The patient may experience hallucinations.
d. The patient must abstain from drinking for 1 week prior to initiating treatment.

83. A group cognitive behavioral therapy (CBT) approach that focuses on relapse prevention for substance use disorders will likely:

a. Stress the importance of attending Alcoholics or Narcotics Anonymous (AA or NA) meetings.
b. Stress mindfulness and accepting oneself.
c. Help patients identify situations that make them vulnerable to relapse.
d. Advise patients to serve as mentors for each other.

84. When developing a plan of care for a patient with bulimia nervosa, the PMHNP includes instructions that state that after the patient finishes eating a meal:

a. The patient must remain seated at the table for 1 hour.
b. An attendant must stay with the patient for 1 hour.
c. The patient must be reminded to avoid purging.
d. The patient must be weighed and measured.

85. A 23-year-old patient complains of multiple physical and mental disorders, including anxiety, irregular menses, neck pain, abdominal cramping, joint pain, frequent and painful urination, headaches, diarrhea, and abdominal distention. Laboratory and radiologic findings have been negative. The PMHNP recognizes these signs and symptoms as probable:

a. Somatic symptom disorder
b. Conversion disorder
c. Illness anxiety disorder
d. Factitious disorder

86. If the patient is in the Precontemplation stage of change regarding cocaine use, according to the Transtheoretical Model (TTM) (Prochaska), the PMHNP recognizes that the initial step in helping him quit using cocaine through a self-help program should be to:

 a. Advise the patient to wait until he is psychologically ready.
 b. Advise the patient to immediately begin the self-help program.
 c. Advise the patient that self-help programs are generally ineffective.
 d. Help the patient progress beyond the stage of Precontemplation.

87. If a patient's electronic health record indicates that she has a negative variance to the clinical pathway, this means that:

 a. The patient has responded more quickly than the projected timeline.
 b. The patient's symptoms are inconsistent with those for which the pathway is intended.
 c. The patient has failed to achieve a desired state on the projected timeline.
 d. The patient expresses negative concerns about the clinical pathway.

88. Considering para-verbal communication, if a person speaks rapidly and loudly in a high-pitched voice, the listener is likely to feel that the speaker is:

 a. Bored with the conversation
 b. Intelligent and deliberate
 c. Confused about the topic of conversation
 d. Angry about something

89. A patient has persistent delusions of persecution. The first step in helping the patient to manage the delusions is to:

 a. Establish a trusting relationship.
 b. Encourage the patient to ignore the delusions.
 c. Instruct the patient in reality testing.
 d. Challenge the patient's sense of reality.

90. According to the DSM-5-TR, a patient could be diagnosed with schizophrenia spectrum if the symptoms are limited to:

 a. Disorganized behavior and negative symptoms
 b. Constant hallucinations (voices judging behavior)
 c. Disorganized speech
 d. Catatonic behavior

91. A patient with generalized anxiety disorder wants to try complementary therapy in addition to medication. The complementary therapy that is most likely to provide some relief of symptoms is:

 a. Aromatherapy
 b. Homeopathy
 c. Relaxation/visualization
 d. Acupuncture

92. An outpatient patient with opioid use disorder is to be maintained on Suboxone (buprenorphine/naloxone). In the induction phase, the PMHNP prescribes:

    a. Suboxone with first administration 24 hours after last short-acting opioid
    b. Suboxone with first administration 12 hours after last long-acting opioid
    c. Suboxone with first administration immediately after last opioid
    d. Suboxone with first administration 12 hours after last short-acting opioid

93. A patient has experienced 2 severe depressive episodes that lasted 4 and 6 weeks, during which he had decreased energy, loss of appetite, insomnia, and suicidal ideation. The patient also had 1 hypomanic episode that lasted about 10 days. The symptoms have interfered with his life, resulting in loss of employment and estrangement from family. The PMHNP knows these symptoms are consistent with:

    a. Bipolar II
    b. Bipolar I
    c. Rapid-cycling bipolar disorder
    d. Cyclothymia

94. The ethnic group that is most likely to believe that neurobiological disorder is the result of a loss of self-control or punishment for bad behavior is:

    a. Mexican American
    b. Japanese American
    c. Puerto Rican
    d. Chinese

95. A patient has been diagnosed with bipolar disorder but has consistently refused to take medications or attend therapy, insisting that he has been misdiagnosed and has only "mild stress." The PMHNP recognizes this patient is probably experiencing:

    a. Dissociation
    b. Resistance
    c. Denial
    d. Suppression

96. If a 35-year-old patient with schizophrenia and paranoia states she does not want her parents (who are paying for her care) to visit because she believes they are "possessed by devils," the PMHNP should:

    a. Ask the physician to intervene.
    b. Allow the parents to visit.
    c. Respect the patient's request.
    d. Suggest the parents get a court order to allow visits.

97. A patient presents with generalized anxiety disorder with rapid onset. Due to the severity of the condition the nurse practitioner prescribes:

    a. Clonazepam
    b. Venlafaxine
    c. Fluoxetine
    d. Buspirone

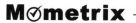

98. An appropriate intervention for a nursing diagnosis of "disturbed thought processes" is:

    a. Encourage the patient to discuss delusions.
    b. Give detailed explanations about unit procedures.
    c. Keep a dim light on during the night to comfort the patient.
    d. Orient the patient to reality frequently and in various ways.

99. If a patient with severe postpartum depression admits she hates her infant but states, "I would never hurt it," the first priority should be to:

    a. Encourage the patient to ask for help with childcare.
    b. Advise the patient's husband to monitor childcare.
    c. Remove the infant from the patient's care.
    d. Advise the patient to find a family member to care for the child.

100. If a family member of a patient asks the PMHNP what constitutes probable cause for involuntary commitment, the best response is:

    a. "You should ask an attorney about that."
    b. "The person is a threat to self or others."
    c. "The person is uncooperative with the family."
    d. "The person is no longer able to work and is homeless."

101. A 50-year-old man with chronic alcoholism presents with increasing confusion, apathy, antegrade and retrograde memory loss, and disorientation, although there is no fever, headache, or laboratory indication of infection. On examination, the PMHNP notes disheveled appearance, malnourishment, ataxia with short gait and wide-based stance, as well as nystagmus and impaired ocular movements. Based on these findings, the nurse practitioner initially prescribes:

    a. Iron for iron deficiency anemia
    b. Cobalamin (vitamin B12) for cobalamin deficiency
    c. Vitamin D and calcium for malnutrition
    d. Thiamine (vitamin B1) for Wernicke-Korsakoff syndrome

102. If a PMHNP knows the employer of a patient and tells the employer that the patient is too mentally unstable to work and the patient loses his job as a result, this may constitute:

    a. Defamation of character
    b. Libel
    c. Invasion of privacy
    d. Battery

103. The most effective method of advocating for the value and role of the PMHNP is to:

    a. Compare achievements to those of other staff members.
    b. Remind staff of the educational preparation required for advanced practice.
    c. Conduct clinical research and present findings to multiple groups.
    d. List achievements at staff meetings and in one-on-one interactions.

104. When working with a patient with conduct disorder, limit setting includes (1) informing the patient of limits, (2) explaining the consequences of noncompliance, and (3):

    a. Providing feedback
    b. Stating reasons
    c. Establishing time limits
    d. Stating expected behaviors

105. A patient receiving cognitive behavioral therapy reports having many automatic thoughts that he is stupid. An appropriate response by the PMHNP is:

    a. "What evidence do you have that you are stupid?"
    b. "You don't appear stupid to me."
    c. "There's always someone smarter than you."
    d. "Why do you think you feel stupid?"

106. The effect of the Medicare prospective payment system on health care has been that a primary concern about patient care is:

    a. Discharge/readmission
    b. Patient satisfaction
    c. Community services
    d. Patient acuity

107. According to the National Quality Forum (NQF), a Serious Reportable Event (SRE) related to *Patient Protection* would include:

    a. A patient is raped by a member of the staff on the hospital grounds.
    b. A patient receives an electric shock from faulty wiring.
    c. A patient dies because of a medical error.
    d. A patient cuts his wrists while hospitalized.

108. A 17-year-old patient with bulimia nervosa has been purging by forcing herself to vomit, taking furosemide (which she stole from her grandmother), and taking OTC laxatives. The electrolyte imbalance that the PMHNP should be most concerned about is:

    a. Hypokalemia
    b. Hyperkalemia
    c. Hypocalcemia
    d. Hypercalcemia

109. A 30-year-old patient whose father sexually abused her showed little emotional response after her father died and expressed relief at his passing but has recently experienced repeated episodes of crying and dreams about her father. The PMHNP recognizes that the type of complicated grief response that the patient is exhibiting is:

    a. Traumatic
    b. Conflicted
    c. Inhibited
    d. Chronic

110. If a 26-year-old female patient with a history of anorexia nervosa has an ideal body weight of 130 pounds, the weight at which the patient will first be diagnosed with a relapse is:

    a. 117 pounds (90% of ideal)
    b. 113 pounds (87% of ideal)
    c. 107 pounds (82% of ideal)
    d. 104 pounds (80% of ideal)

111. A 19-year-old patient with schizophrenia has not responded to conventional antipsychotics and is having increasing episodes of violence toward his parents, with whom he lives, and has persistent suicidal ideation, so the PMHNP plans to switch the patient to clozapine (Clozaril). For the next 6 months the PMHNP will expect to monitor:

    a. Weekly white blood cell counts
    b. Monthly red blood cell counts
    c. Weekly platelet counts
    d. Weekly serum glucose

112. When helping the family of a patient develop a crisis safety plan, an approach that is appropriate to use as a de-escalation technique is:

    a. Take control of the situation.
    b. Attempt to reason with the patient.
    c. Touch the person on the arm or hand to defuse his or her tension.
    d. Quietly describe any action before carrying it out.

113. A patient who complains that the doctor implanted a controlling microchip in his arm and that he needs to cut it out is experiencing a:

    a. Somatic delusion
    b. Nihilistic delusion
    c. Delusion of control
    d. Delusion of persecution

114. A 65-year-old man with frontotemporal dementia has increasing problems communicating with difficulty both understanding and producing language. The type of aphasia that is most common to frontotemporal dementia is:

    a. Broca's aphasia
    b. Primary progressive aphasia
    c. Anomic aphasia
    d. Wernicke's aphasia

115. When developing an education plan for a group of homeless patients with alcohol use disorder, the most important information to include is probably information about:

    a. Community resources
    b. Inpatient facilities
    c. Personal responsibility
    d. Medications to control alcohol use disorder

116. The most common reason for nonadherence to medical treatment for a neurobiological disorder is that the patient:

a. Has double diagnosis with drug or alcohol use disorder
b. Dislikes adverse effects of medications
c. Is too confused to take medications
d. Does not believe he or she has a neurobiological disorder

117. The PMHNP has suggested a change in procedure based on evidence-based research but has encountered considerable staff resistance. The best approach is to:

a. Advise staff that they should cooperate and be open to change.
b. Suggest a limited trial period to evaluate the effect of the change.
c. Ask the administration to require the change.
d. Withdraw the suggestion.

118. The most common comorbid condition associated with schizophrenia is:

a. Panic disorder
b. Post-traumatic stress disorder
c. Substance use disorder
d. Obsessive-compulsive disorder

119. If a patient is engaged in injection drug use, the PMHNP should advise the patient to receive vaccinations for:

a. Hepatitis C
b. HIV/AIDS
c. Herpes zoster
d. Hepatitis A and hepatitis B

120. A 17-year-old patient has been diagnosed with Tourette's syndrome. As part of a complete examination, the PMHNP should assess the patient for the common comorbidities of:

a. ADHD and obsessive-compulsive disorder
b. Depression and obsessive-compulsive disorder
c. Schizophrenia
d. ADHD and autism spectrum disorder

121. During the initial clinical interview, the patient states repeatedly that his boss is to blame for all of the patient's problems and that the boss "is going to pay." The PMHNP should respond by asking:

a. "Why do you feel that way?"
b. "What thoughts have you had about hurting your boss?"
c. "Can you think of other reasons for your problems?"
d. "Do you think that this anger toward your boss is productive?"

122. A patient with panic disorder has been successfully controlled with alprazolam (Xanax) but has recently developed signs of CNS depression, including lethargy, drowsiness, confusion, lack of coordination, bradycardia, and bradypnea. Following a positive tuberculosis test, the patient was started on isoniazid prophylaxis 2 weeks earlier and also takes hydrochlorothiazide for mild hypertension. The most likely cause of the CNS depression is:

    a. Combination of a CYP3A4 substrate (alprazolam) with an inhibitor (isoniazid)
    b. Combination of a CYP3A4 substrate (alprazolam) with an inducer (isoniazid)
    c. Combination of a CYP2D6 substrate (hydrochlorothiazide) with an inhibitor (alprazolam)
    d. Combination of a CYP2D6 substrate (isoniazid) with an inducer (hydrochlorothiazide)

123. If an aggressive, hostile patient has managed to remove a towel rod and is brandishing it as a weapon, the PMHNP's first priority should be to:

    a. Disarm the patient
    b. Subdue the patient
    c. Protect self and others
    d. Leave the patient's immediate environment

124. A 34-year-old male patient who returned from military service in Afghanistan has begun to have severe frightening flashbacks related to post-traumatic stress disorder (PTSD). If the PMHNP finds the patient cowering in the corner of the room in a state of panic, the best approach is to say:

    a. "Give me your hand and I'll help you up."
    b. "I know you are afraid, but you are safe here."
    c. "Just breathe deeply and relax."
    d. "There is nothing to be afraid of."

125. A mother brings a 2-year-old child to see the PMHNP, describing a pattern of developmental delays, increasing tantrums, and failure of the child to interact with others. During the visit, the child holds his hands close to his face and focuses on the movement of his fingers, ignoring the nurse practitioner and his mother and avoiding eye contact. The screening test that the nurse practitioner should initially recommend is:

    a. Vision test
    b. IQ test
    c. Hearing test
    d. The modified checklist for autism in toddlers (M-CHAT-R)

126. A 22-year-old Asian patient who is intolerant of alcohol tells the PMHNP that a friend has advised him that he can avoid flushing and drink alcohol without symptoms if he takes an H2 blocker, such as ranitidine or famotidine, before drinking. The best response is:

    a. This is a safe method of improving tolerance to alcohol.
    b. This can result in alcohol poisoning.
    c. This only works if the medications are taken every 4 hours.
    d. These medications have no effect.

127. Considering Maslow's hierarchy, the order in which the following nursing diagnoses for a patient should be prioritized (first to last) is:

a. (1) deficient fluid volume, (2) risk for self-injury, (3) sexual dysfunction, and (4) low self-esteem

b. (1) low self-esteem, (2) risk for self-injury, (3) deficient fluid volume, and (4) sexual dysfunction

c. (1) deficient fluid volume, (2) low self-esteem, (3) risk for self-injury, and (4) sexual dysfunction

d. (1) risk for self-injury, (2) deficient fluid volume, (3) sexual dysfunction, and (4) low self-esteem

128. The primary risk factor for alcohol abuse and dependence is:

a. Genetic predisposition
b. Peer influence
c. Gender
d. Socioeconomic status

129. In milieu therapy ("therapeutic community"), if a person exhibits inappropriate behavior, the correct response is to:

a. Ignore the behavior.
b. Ask the other patients to determine consequences.
c. Help the patient examine the effect the behavior has on others.
d. Apply punishment or restrictions for the inappropriate behavior.

130. The PMHNP is conducting research as part of evidence-based practice and is reading research reviews. The nurse practitioner must recognize that the most subjective type of review is:

a. Integrative
b. Narrative
c. Systematic
d. Meta-analysis

131. If a patient is being evaluated for depression and laboratory results show that the patient's free T4 level is 0.6 ng/dL (normal 0.8-1.5 ng/dL) and the thyroid-stimulating hormone (TSH) level is 7.4 mIU/L (normal 0.4-4.0 mIU/L), this suggests that depression:

a. May result from hypoparathyroidism related to pituitary dysfunction
b. May result from hypothyroidism related to thyroid dysfunction
c. May result from hyperparathyroidism related to thyroid dysfunction
d. Is likely unrelated to thyroid dysfunction

132. Patients taking lithium for bipolar disorder are likely to begin to exhibit signs of toxicity if levels exceed:

a. 0.5 mEq/L
b. 0.8 mEq/L
c. 1.0 mEq/L
d. 1.5 mEq/L

133. When conducting research using a database search for evidence-based practice, the PMHNP should avoid:

   a. Truncations
   b. Wildcards
   c. Stopwords
   d. Nesting

134. When conducting a physical examination of a patient, the PMHNP notes a flattening of the patient's nasolabial fold and drooping of the lower eyelids, suggesting injury to the:

   a. 4th cranial nerve
   b. 5th cranial nerve
   c. 6th cranial nerve
   d. 7th cranial nerve

135. The PMHNP is evaluating an outpatient who states repeatedly that he wants to die. The question that is most critical is:

   a. "Do you have access to dangerous weapons?"
   b. "Can you stay with family or friends?"
   c. "What can I do to help you?"
   d. "Why do you feel this way?"

136. The PMHNP recognizes that the first essential element in providing trauma-informed care is to:

   a. Ask all patients if they have experienced trauma.
   b. Recognize the prevalence of trauma and its effects.
   c. Recognize that trauma experiences are similar for most patients.
   d. View trauma through a narrow lens, focusing only on trauma events.

137. If a 12-year-old child is diagnosed with conduct disorder, a behavior that indicates that the child is at risk of progress to antisocial personality disorder includes:

   a. Episodes of depression
   b. Occasional lying
   c. Substance abuse
   d. Cruelty to animals

138. All of the following domains are assessed with the Denver Developmental Screening Test II (DDST-II) for young children except:

   a. Language
   b. Gross motor
   c. Cognitive
   d. Personal-social

139. The PMHNP believes that an additional staff member should be hired for the psychiatric unit and plans to take the request to administration, but the administration usually turns down such requests, citing inadequate financial resources. The most appropriate action for the nurse practitioner is to:

    a. Reorganize existing staff.
    b. Prepare a cost-benefit analysis.
    c. Gather signatures in support of the request.
    d. Threaten to resign if the request is denied.

140. A 6-year-old child who is hospitalized with a serious illness has been very withdrawn and is drawing a picture of a boy in a bed crying, with large tears on the face falling onto the pillows. The most appropriate statement to elicit the child's feelings is:

    a. "Why is the little boy in your picture crying?"
    b. "Is the little boy afraid to be in the hospital?"
    c. "I see that the little boy in your picture is crying."
    d. "Did something hurt the little boy?"

141. The PMHNP is observing an interdisciplinary team to determine what works and what does not work. The nurse practitioner notes a number of negative practices, including:

    a. Members interrupt speakers and interpret their comments.
    b. Members ask clarifying questions after another member speaks.
    c. Members react to facts rather than feelings.
    d. Members avoid giving unsolicited advice.

142. If the PMHNP plans to access the healthcare system's data warehouse for research purposes, this is referred to as:

    a. Accessing
    b. Keying
    c. Data mining
    d. Drilling down

143. According to Gestalt therapy (Perls), the term for a boundary disturbance that involves accepting the beliefs/opinions of other people without questioning them is:

    a. Projection
    b. Retroflection
    c. Deflection
    d. Introjection

144. Conflicts have arisen between the PMHNP and an administrator regarding policies. They have agreed to discuss their disagreements in a non-binding semi-formal process assisted by the director of human resources. This type of alternative dispute resolution is:

    a. Arbitration
    b. Mediation
    c. Collaboration
    d. Compromise

145. If the PMHNP determines that a patient who is confused and hallucinating is at risk for self-injury and must have a sitter, but the patient refuses the sitter, who stays despite the patient's refusal, this demonstrates a situation in which the ethical principle of autonomy is in conflict with the principle of:

    a. Nonmaleficence
    b. Verity
    c. Beneficence
    d. Justice

146. A patient describes a number of failures in her life, including loss of employment, divorce, estrangement from family members, and financial difficulties. The response by the PMHNP that exemplifies reflection is:

    a. "Can you tell me more about your feelings about these events?"
    b. "You feel sad because of all the disappointments in your life."
    c. "What steps could you take to improve your situation?"
    d. "It sounds as though you have been disappointed many times."

147. The first step in successfully communicating within and across an organization in order to promote change is to:

    a. Identify key concerns of different individuals/departments.
    b. Make a plan regarding communication.
    c. Outline the steps to change for all individuals/departments.
    d. Ask for input in how to communicate.

148. If utilizing the FOCUS (find, organize, clarify, uncover, start) model of performance improvement, the initial step is to find:

    a. Key stakeholders in bringing about change
    b. The underlying reasons for problems
    c. What is working well in the organization
    d. What is not working well in the organization

149. When determining sample size for evidence-based inquiry, according to the "Rule of 10," if the variables being studied for a sample population included (1) age, (2) gender, (3) education, and (4) marital status, the minimum number of subjects required is:

    a. 10
    b. 40
    c. 50
    d. 20

150. In keeping with professional standards, if the PMHNP wants to become a political activist, an appropriate form of activism would be to:

    a. Discuss political concerns with patients.
    b. Post political posters in the workplace.
    c. Write letters/emails to politicians regarding concerns.
    d. Question workplace associates about their political beliefs.

151. In the hospital where the PMHNP is employed, the psychiatric unit, the suicide hotline, the outpatient substance abuse program, the program for homeless veterans, and a community mental health clinic as well as the psychiatric assessment team in the emergency department are all under the management of the same executive. This type of organizational structure is referred to as:

   a. Service-line
   b. Functional
   c. Matrix
   d. Flat

152. A patient with borderline personality disorder tells the PMHNP that she has a secret and will tell the nurse practitioner only if the nurse practitioner promises not to tell the others on the mental health team. The most appropriate response is:

   a. "I promise I won't tell the others, so your secret is safe with me."
   b. "You're just trying to manipulate me, so I don't want to hear it."
   c. "You have the right to decide what information I can share."
   d. "I can't keep information regarding your health or well-being from other team members."

153. The PMHNP is evaluating an increasingly withdrawn 8-year-old child who was injured in a motor vehicle accident that killed his mother. The practitioner knows the best approach is to:

   a. Avoid discussing the traumatic event directly.
   b. Reassure the child that everything will be all right.
   c. Remind the child that his father is still alive.
   d. Talk to the child about the traumatic event.

154. The PMHNP is to lead an interprofessional team that includes nurses, a physician, a social worker, a rehabilitation therapist, a dietician, and an occupational therapist. The first thing the nurse practitioner should do in preparation for leadership is to:

   a. Develop a hierarchical system, indicating which members are most important.
   b. Inform the team members of procedures for team meetings.
   c. Study team members' job descriptions and learn their roles and responsibilities.
   d. Inform team members of goals for working together cooperatively.

155. The PMHNP was instrumental in establishing a population-based public health intervention program for at-risk youth and has developed a series of workshops, posters, and pamphlets regarding the dangers of drug and alcohol abuse. This type of prevention effort is:

   a. Primary
   b. Secondary
   c. Tertiary
   d. Quaternary

156. A patient with borderline personality disorder is most likely to benefit from:

   a. Cognitive behavioral therapy
   b. Psychoanalysis
   c. Milieu therapy
   d. Dialectical behavioral therapy

157. When conducting gap analysis as part of the quality improvement process, the first step is to:

    a. Identify gaps between current processes and goals.
    b. Assess current situations/processes.
    c. Identify resources.
    d. Outline process required to achieve target outcomes.

158. The PMHNP is conducting a psychiatric exam. Homicidal, suicidal, and violent ideations are evaluated in order to assess the element of:

    a. Judgment and insight
    b. Thought process
    c. Abnormal/psychotic thoughts
    d. Mood and affect

159. A three-and-a-half-year-old child is potty trained for urination but insists on wearing a diaper for bowel movements. The child's mother asks the PMHNP for guidance. The nurse practitioner suggests:

    a. Using incentives or disincentives
    b. Punishing the child by taking away toys
    c. Making the child wear diapers all of the time
    d. Telling the child that diapers are for babies

160. When trying to help patients reduce risk factors, such as drinking and smoking, for which there is little immediate reward, the PMHNP should assist the patient to:

    a. Focus on personal rewards of achievement.
    b. Keep focused on health rewards.
    c. Establish short-term and long-term goals.
    d. Make lists of reasons to reduce risks.

161. The PMHNP is educating a patient and family about neuroplasticity following a traumatic brain injury (TBI). The nurse practitioner accurately provides education that the patient should:

    a. Take medications to alter brain chemistry.
    b. Do relaxation exercises and visualization.
    c. Imagine carrying out physical activities.
    d. Do repetitive physical exercises/activities.

162. According to Kohlberg's theory of moral development, the stage at which a 9-year-old child may make moral judgments based on what the child gets from the decision is:

    a. Punishment and obedience orientation
    b. Instrumental relativist orientation
    c. Interpersonal concordance
    d. Law and order orientation

163. If the PMHNP wants to effect health policy, he or she should begin by gaining information about the:

    a. System (local, state, federal)
    b. Specific issues of interest
    c. Key stakeholders
    d. Processes involved

164. An organizational structure in which professional and non-professional staff members are divided according to the type of work that they do (nursing, laboratory, housekeeping) and staff report to discipline specific managers is classified as:

    a. Matrix
    b. Parallel
    c. Functional
    d. Program

165. The PMHNP is testing the reliability of 2 staff members' scoring in a research project by having them measure the same event together and then comparing their scores. This method tests for:

    a. Stability
    b. Internal consistency
    c. External consistency
    d. Equivalence

166. As supervisor in the psychiatric unit, the PMHNP often presents decisions and welcomes staff members to give input and to pose questions, although the nurse practitioner rarely changes decisions. This leadership style is:

    a. Participative
    b. Consultative
    c. Democratic
    d. Autocratic

167. When assigning roles to team members, the PMHNP should first consider their:

    a. Personality types
    b. Education and skills
    c. Commitment to team efforts
    d. Available time investment

168. An example of shared governance is:

    a. Unit teams establish work schedules for their own units.
    b. Administrators receive regular reports of executive decisions.
    c. The administration allows incentive pay for 12-hour shifts.
    d. Units are rewarded for achieving cost-cutting goals.

169. The PMHNP in a psychiatric unit notes that nursing staff members often seem very surprised when patients are discharged. This is probably an indication of:

    a. Staff incompetence
    b. Staff turnover
    c. Different goals
    d. Poor communication

170. The PMHNP is assigned as care manager for a group of patients. The first task the nurse practitioner should complete is:

a. Care plans
b. Staff assignments
c. Needs assessments
d. Cost analysis

171. The administration has mandated a change in procedure as a cost-cutting measure, resulting in both active and passive resistance. An example of passive resistance is:

a. Agreeing but failing to act
b. Verbally attacking the change
c. Organizing resistance
d. Refusing the make the change

172. In a psychiatric unit, patients are primarily able to exercise power through:

a. Threats and intimidation
b. Praise and complaints
c. Cooperation/lack of cooperation
d. Rewards and punishments

173. A newly hired PMHNP routinely stays after work (unpaid) to review records and care plans and make sure that everything is properly documented and thorough. During the performance review, the supervisor is likely to note that the nurse practitioner needs improvement in:

a. Competence
b. Care management
c. Confidence
d. Time management

174. The PMHNP has become supervisor of the neurobiology unit. The practice has been that every nurse on the unit be assigned the same number of patients, but lower reimbursement has resulted in a loss of 2 positions. The best solution for assigning patients is to:

a. Divide the patients equally among the remaining staff.
b. Ask the staff how they would like to manage the problem.
c. Switch to an acuity-based model.
d. Demand that the administration authorize additional hiring.

175. The PMHNP notes that team members seem to have difficulty with time management. The best method of dealing with this is to begin with:

a. A discussion about time management
b. A time log for a week
c. More specific assignments
d. A survey regarding needs

Answers and Explanations

1. D: This is an example of groupthink. Groupthink occurs when maintaining the status quo is more important to members of a group than making a reasoned or good decision.

2. C: An effective method of handling diversity in the workplace is to develop internal support systems. Diversity should be recognized and valued rather than acting as though everyone is alike because that standard usually means that people are expected to conform to the prevailing majority culture/group. It is important to ensure all individuals are treated in a fair manner. Problems related to diversity can rarely be solved quickly, so dealing with diversity must be an ongoing process rather than a once-a-year diversity workshop.

3. B: If the NP works in a community in which many people are uninsured or underinsured, the impact on health care is most likely that many of these people will postpone health care until a crisis occurs. This often results in more expensive care and greater need for care. Being uninsured or underinsured is most often associated with low socioeconomic status, which tends to translate to low power, meaning that the people are less able to organize.

4. A: Population-based interventions are aimed at vulnerable or underserved subgroups within the larger population. For example, a program may be tailored to the needs of an immigrant population or the homeless. These subgroups often have health disparities and need both health care for existing problems and preventive measures to prevent illness. Population-based programs should improve access to quality care and meet unmet healthcare needs at no or low costs to encourage utilization of services.

5. D: The NP should help this patient to identify other support systems because patients often view support from a narrow perspective. Support systems may include other family members, neighbors, friends, religious organizations, support groups, and community agencies.

6. A: From the perspective of risk management, an incident that would be classified as a serious incident includes a patient falling and spraining her wrist. Serious incidents include interruptions of treatment and minor injuries that would not require hospitalization. Service occurrences include minor damage to equipment or property and inadequate provision of care (usually related to patient complaints). Sentinel events involve unexpected death or permanent physical or psychological injury and include suicide and rape.

7. C: Communication. The 3 primary components of risk analysis are:

- Assessment: gathering and analyzing data through a variety of means.
- Intervention: using data to make changes in order to reduce risk.
- Communication: publishing/sharing results with various key stakeholders, including administration, staff, patients, families, and the general public.
- Risk analysis may be carried out to assess individual risks as well as risks associated with different treatments or programs. All new treatments and/or programs should undergo risk assessment.

8. A: This type of testing is convergent testing. If there is no positive correlation, then a different instrument may be needed or the screening parameters changed.

9. B: The premise of servant leadership is that the leader is not meant to simply exercise power and make decisions but to serve all those within the organization and/or community. Leadership is considered an altruistic endeavor. Thus, essential qualities of a servant leader include the ability to listen effectively to the input of others and to exercise empathy, always putting the organizational needs and greater good above personal needs. The leader needs to have a good sense of self-awareness and the ability to persuade and influence others.

10. D: The Health Insurance Portability and Accountability Act (HIPAA, 1996) privacy rules allow unrestricted disclosure only of patients' de-identified health information, usually aggregated for purposes of research. Health information may be de-identified by a formal determination by a qualified statistician, or through removal of specific identifiers such as the name of the patient, family members, household members, and employers, as well as date of birth, Social Security number, other ID number, telephone number, and address.

11. D: The National Institute of Mental Health collects a wealth of data. The 4 primary categories of data include:

- Prevalence: subcategories include serious mental health illness by demographics (age, sex, race), specific disorders, use of services and treatment, and specific populations (such as inmates).
- Disability: subcategories include disability and years of life lost.
- Suicide: subcategories include rates, suicidality, and causes of death.
- Cost: subcategories include estimates, payers, receivers, trends, and comparisons (among the 5 most expensive medical conditions, which include heart conditions, cancer, trauma-related conditions, asthma, as well as mental disorders).

12. A: When faced with an ethical dilemma in caring for a patient, the PMHNP should share concerns with others, such as an ethics committee, in order to reach a resolution. Personal bias can make trying to reach a conclusion independently difficult, as people are often unaware of their biases. Most organizations have ethics committees that are trained to deal with ethical issues. Trying to ignore an issue or to resolve it with the help of a close friend (who may not be unbiased because of the relationship) are not good solutions.

13. C: If a patient with end-stage renal disease is confused and delusional, the nursing diagnosis that should be entered in the plan of care is disturbed thought processes. With end-stage renal disease, the body is unable to clear toxins from the blood. A number of factors can contribute to mental confusion, including hypertension (which can cause cerebral ischemia), electrolyte imbalance (hyperkalemia, hypernatremia, hyperphosphatemia, and hypocalcemia), and acid-base disturbance (which results in nervous system dysfunction).

14. B: Dystonic reactions (spasms of the eye, neck, tongue, back, and other muscles) are common during early stages of treatment with antipsychotics, especially high-potency drugs administered parenterally and in high doses. The reactions may occur immediately or be delayed for a few hours or days. Dystonic reactions are rare after the first 3 months of treatment. The reactions usually subside with the administration of IM diphenhydramine followed by oral administration. Benztropine may also be used to treat dystonic reactions.

15. A: In a therapeutic milieu, the primary action of the PMHNP in helping patients to develop effective interpersonal skills is role modeling. The nurse practitioner models behavior that supports appropriate boundaries and helps patients learn appropriate responses. Interpersonal skills include showing respect, caring, managing conflicts, and being assertive, genuine, and honest. For example, if a patient is asked to introduce himself but states he is uncomfortable talking, the nurse practitioner might model acceptance by stating: "I appreciate your trying."

16. D: When conducting examinations of patients, the PMHNP should keep in mind that the psychiatric diagnosis for which there are the most differential diagnoses is generalized anxiety disorder (as well as other anxiety disorders). Symptoms of anxiety are often very nonspecific and may occur in a multitude of other psychiatric and nonpsychiatric disorders, and may also occur with drug toxicity and drug withdrawal. Many medications, including corticosteroids and bronchodilators, may cause anxiety.

17. B: When using the LEARN (listen, explain, acknowledge, recommend, negotiate) model for cross-cultural health care, an important approach to the Explain step is to use drawings, videos, and test results to demonstrate the information the PMHNP is trying to convey. Providing concrete information/demonstrations helps patients to better understand, especially when cultural differences result in perceptions of illness that may be at odds with Western beliefs.

18. C: When addressing a group of older adults at a senior citizens' center about mental health, the neuroprotective strategy that the PMHNP should recommend as valuable for almost all older adults is physical exercise. Exercise promotes neuroplasticity and brain functioning. Patients should also be encouraged to stay mentally active, such as through learning new skills and doing mental exercises (such as Sudoku).

19. D: For various reasons, some people may be excluded from a study so that instead of randomized subjects, the subjects may be highly selected; therefore, when data which have internal validity are compared with data of another population in which there is less or more selection, results may be different. The selection of subjects, in this case, would interfere with external validity. Part of the design of a study should include considerations of whether or not it should have external validity or whether there is value for the institution based solely on internal validation.

20. B: The ECG change that should be monitored with risperidone is a prolonged QT segment. If this occurs, the patient may require an alternative medication. Other cardiovascular adverse effects associated with antipsychotics include postural hypotension (most common with low-potency antipsychotics) and arrhythmias and palpitations (associated with higher doses and combinations of drugs). Patients on antipsychotics should have routine monitoring of cardiovascular status, including an ECG.

21. B: If the PMHNP is conducting a problem-focused office visit with an established patient in order to titrate medication, the number of elements of the psychiatric exam that must be included for CMS billing purposes is 1-5. Elements of the psychiatric exam include speech, thought processes, associations, abnormal/psychotic thoughts, judgment/insights, orientation, recent and remote memory, attention and concentration language, fund of knowledge, and mood and affect.

22. C: The response that has the highest priority is "Are you thinking about killing yourself?" Suicidal ideation is common when people are distraught and overwhelmed and feel their situations are "hopeless," so this should be addressed directly.

23. A: According to Kotter's model for organizational change, the first phase involves establishing a sense of urgency. The primary means of establishing urgency is to draw attention to a problem through the collection and dissemination of data. Then, a coalition needs to be formed of individuals sharing similar goals. This group develops a vision for change and communicates the vision to others. Next, individuals must be empowered to make changes, meaning that they have responsibilities as well as accountabilities. Short-term gains should be recognized in order to reinforce change and then gains consolidated and increased. Anchoring change, ensuring it will persist, is the last phase.

24. D: Coercion. Sources of power in an organization usually derive from:

1. Authority: usually related to position in the hierarchy (administrator, supervisor, team leader)
2. Reward: usually derived from administrator and supervisors and include increased salary, benefits, and recognition
3. Expertise: special knowledge that sets an individual apart and allows the person to exercise some degree of authority, such as a PMHNP
4. Coercion: the ability to require others to do or say something, such as occurs when a manager makes an assignment or passes judgment

25. D: The cytochrome P450 enzyme that metabolizes approximately 50% of current drugs is CYP3A4. Many commonly used medications, such as alprazolam (Xanax), sildenafil (Viagra), and carbamazepine (Tegretol), are CYP3A4 substrates. However, many other common drugs are CYP450 inhibitors or inducers, which affect the metabolism of the substrates. If a substrate is given in conjunction with an inhibitor, the metabolism of the substrate is slowed, allowing drug levels to increase to toxic levels. If a substrate is given with an inducer, metabolism of the substrate increases, resulting in an inadequate blood level.

26. C: The initial step in resolving this problem should be to decrease the dosage of the SSRI because the symptoms are often dose-related. However, it may take a few weeks at a lower dosage before improvement is seen. If this is unsuccessful, the next step is to try a different antidepressant, such as an SSRI with a lower rate of sexual side effects or a different class of antidepressant. Antidotes, such as sildenafil or bethanechol, may be useful for some patients.

27. B: Distribution: The volume of distribution is the relationship between the total loading dose of drug administered and the serum concentration (volume of body fluid required to dissolve the amount of drug found in the serum). Absorption: This relates to the rate at which a drug enters the bloodstream and the amount of drug. Metabolism: Drug transformation that makes it hydrophilic enough to be eliminated. Clearance: Elimination pathways (liver, kidney) can become saturated if the dose is too high or administration is too frequent. Ideally, a drug concentration should be maintained at a steady state (average).

28. A: When disseminating evidence regarding adverse effects associated with a medication to a large number of patients and families in a widespread area, the best method is likely regular mail in addition to an email notice to make sure that the message is received. With large numbers of patients, telephone calls may be too time consuming, especially because many people screen calls so the call goes to voicemail. Personal visits are usually not practical, and group meetings put the burden on the patient to attend.

29. C: The cardiac enzyme test that is most diagnostic is troponin I. Troponin I and T are both found in the cardiac muscle and are released when the heart muscle is damaged. However, troponin I is specific to the heart. Troponin levels begin to increase within 3-6 hours of cardiac damage with troponin I, peaking in 14-20 hours. Troponin T peaks within 12-24 hours.

30. D: The most appropriate study design is a cohort study. The cohort study is an observational study that follows groups over a period of time to determine the incidence of a problem or the relationship between a variable and an outcome.

31. C: The FDA's 21 CFR Parts 50 and 56 regulate protection of human subjects and state that any researcher involving patients in research must obtain informed consent, in language understandable to the patient or the patient's agent. The elements of this informed consent must include an explanation of the research, the purpose, and the expected duration, as well as a description of any potential risks. Potential benefits must be described as well as possible alternative treatments. Any compensation must be outlined. The extent of confidentiality should be clarified.

32. A: While all of these elements are important, best practices identified through literature review should carry the most weight when developing evidence-based guidelines. Preferences are often based on subjective rather than objective observations, and may relate to familiarity and ease of use. Cost-effectiveness is always an issue and must be considered, but it should not be the primary concern. In some cases, spending more to prevent a problem initially may save money in terms of morbidity and extended medical care in the long term.

33. B: The screening test has high sensitivity because it correctly identified most patients (96%) with the condition being measured (noncompliance) with a low rate of false-negatives; however, a rate of 25% false-positives among the compliant group indicates the test has low specificity. High-sensitivity tests have low rates of false-negatives, and low-sensitivity tests have high rates of false-negatives. High-specificity tests have low rates of false-positives, and low-specificity tests have high rates of false-positives.

34. D: There is a fine line between social interactions and interactions that promote a therapeutic alliance between the patient and the mental health nurse practitioner. An example of an interaction that promotes a therapeutic alliance is the patient and nurse practitioner discussing goal setting for the patient. The PMHNP must always be aware of professional boundaries and should avoid sharing mutual experiences, discussing random topics, and maintaining secrets, as these base the relationship on friendship rather than on the patient's need for treatment.

35. C: The nurse practitioner should arrange for a translator. Children should never be used as translators as they lack vocabulary and understanding about health matters and may not interpret correctly. Other adult family members, such as the wife, should not be asked to answer questions for the patient unless the patient is unable to answer questions because of a health condition; a spouse may not understand medical terms and may not translate correctly. Additionally, the patient may have kept information from the family.

36. A: The most essential protective strategy for the PMHNP to employ to reduce the risk of legal action is to meet or exceed the standard of care. The nurse practitioner must be competent and up-to-date with the latest treatments. The nurse practitioner should also be knowledgeable about the state's nurse practice act and the scope and standards of practice, the ANA's code of ethics, and the organization's policies and procedures.

37. B: Because the patient has been taking lorazepam and has a history of narcotic use, the nurse practitioner should suspect coingestion, especially since the patient is exhibiting alternations in consciousness and respiratory depression. In this case, charcoal, concentrated dextrose, thiamine, and naloxone are indicated. Gastric emptying is indicated only if ingestion occurred less than 1 hour ago. Flumazenil (antagonist) 0.2 mg/minute to a total dose of 3 mg may be used in some cases but is not routinely advised because of complications related to benzodiazepine dependency or coingestion of cyclic antidepressants. Flumazenil is contraindicated in the presence of increased intracranial pressure.

38. A: If the PMHNP notes that a patient with frontotemporal dementia has difficulty with executive functioning, this suggests damage to the prefrontal cortex, which lies behind the forehead. Executive functions include the ability to plan, establish goals, and regulate behavior. Patients may have lack of impulse control and the ability to suppress socially unacceptable speech or behavior as well as impaired short-term memory and lack of empathy for others.

39. D: Autonomy is the ethical principle that the individual has the right to make decisions about his or her own care. The nurse practitioner must keep the patients fully informed so they can exercise autonomy in informed decision making. Beneficence is an ethical principle that involves performing actions that are for the purpose of benefitting another person. Nonmaleficence is an ethical principle that means healthcare workers should provide care in a manner that does not cause direct, intentional harm to the patient. Justice is the ethical principle that relates to the distribution of the limited resources of healthcare benefits to the members of society.

40. C: A person's experience with learning can vary widely and is affected by his or her ability to cope with changes, personal goals, motivation to learn, and cultural background. People may have widely divergent ideas about what constitutes illness and/or treatment. Lack of English skills may make learning difficult and prevent people from asking questions. The patient/family's readiness to learn should be assessed because if they are not ready, instruction is of little value. Often readiness is indicated when the patients/families ask questions or show an interest in procedures.

41. A: An action or intervention that may be viewed as retraumatization includes using a confrontational approach in the group. This may be especially traumatizing to victims of abuse. Patients should be encouraged to participate in treatment plans, and screening should be done before a patient is admitted to a group because failing to do so may result in retraumatization. Rules of conduct in the group should be enforced consistently to reduce anxiety among group members.

42. C: Compromise.

Compromise	Both parties make concessions, but this can result in decisions that suit no one, so compromise is not always ideal.
Accommodation	One party concedes to the other, but the losing side may gain little or nothing, so this approach should be used when there is clear benefit to one choice.
Avoidance	When both parties dislike conflict, they may put off negotiating and resolve nothing.
Collaboration	Both parties receive what they want, often through creative solutions, but collaboration may be ineffective with highly competitive parties.
Competition	One party wins and the other loses, sometimes resulting in conflict.

43. A: According to the general adaptation syndrome (Selye) (which comprises alarm, resistance, and exhaustion), an example of reaction to stress in the resistance stage is levels of neurotransmitters and hormones return to normal. The first stage, alarm, includes the fight or flight response with activation of the hormonal, neurotransmitter, and cardiovascular systems. This stage may last for 1 minute to several hours. During the second stage, resistance, the body tries to recover the normal status of the cardiovascular, hormonal, and neurotransmitter systems. If resistance is inadequate, the last stage, exhaustion, can occur, leading to chronic illnesses.

44. D: Suicide gesture: Actions that do not result in harm to the individual who does not actually desire or plan to die. Suicide gestures are often carried out in an attempt to gain attention. Suicide ideation: Thoughts or fantasies about committing suicide accompanied by intent. Suicide threat: Verbal or written statements of the intent to commit suicide. Suicide attempt: Actual actions taken to commit suicide, resulting in minor or major injury or threat to health.

45. A: If a patient's cranial MRI indicates significant atrophy of the hippocampus, the PMHNP should expect that the patient will have the inability to form new long-term memories. However, the patient may be able to retrieve already existing long-term memories (such as those of childhood) and may be able to form short-term memories, such as recalling an appointment time or medication directions for a brief period.

46. B: Category IB. Categories include:

- Category IA: well supported by evidence from experimental, clinical, or epidemiologic studies and strongly recommended for implementation.
- Category IB: supporting evidence from some studies, good theoretical basis, and strongly recommended for implementation.
- Category IC: required by state or federal regulations or an industry standard
- Category II: supported by suggestive clinical or epidemiologic studies, has a theoretical basis, and is suggested for implementation.
- Category III: supported by descriptive studies and may be useful.
- Category IV: obtained from expert opinion or authorities only.
- Unresolved: no recommendation because of a lack of consensus or evidence.

47. D: "I'd like to hear how you feel about that" is an example of therapeutic communication that allows a patient to explore a topic. Nontherapeutic communication includes:

- Meaningless clichés: "Don't worry. Everything will be fine." or "Isn't it a nice day?"
- Providing advice: "You should…" or "The best thing to do is…" When patients ask for advice, it is better to provide facts and encourage the patient to reach a decision.
- Asking for an explanation of behavior that is not directly related to patient care and requires analysis and explanation of feelings: "Why are you so upset?"

48. A: As part of the normal aging process, changes in neurotransmitters usually occur, including decreased levels of serotonin. Serotonin, which is produced in the brainstem and found throughout the brain, helps to regulate body temperature, eating and sleeping patterns, and mood. Inadequate serotonin is associated with depression. Selective serotonin reuptake inhibitors (SSRIs) specifically target serotonin and prevent its reuptake so that more serotonin is available to function as a neurotransmitter.

49. A: When treating anxiety in a geriatric patient, short-acting benzodiazepines, such as lorazepam or temazepam, are usually well tolerated while tricyclic antidepressants and β-adrenergic agents may cause adverse effects. Short-acting benzodiazepines are also the drugs of choice for pediatric patients. Long-acting benzodiazepines may result in confusion in elderly patients. If benzodiazepines are not effective, some people may respond to SSRIs or low-dose antihistamines (especially with respiratory dysfunction). Younger adults may benefit from a wider range of drugs, including both long- and short-acting benzodiazepines, tricyclic antidepressants, and β-adrenergic agents.

50. D: The NP should expect that the patient will require a lower dosage than normal. The components of tobacco smoke affect liver enzymes, often speeding up metabolism and resulting in the need for a higher dose to achieve the same serum level. If the patient stops smoking, then dosages often need to be adjusted downward.

51. C: A number of different types of outcomes data must be considered:

- Integrative: This includes measures of mortality, longevity, and cost-effectiveness.
- Clinical: This includes symptoms, diagnoses, staging of disease, and those indicators of individual health.
- Physiological: This includes measures of physical abnormalities, loss of function, and activities of daily living.
- Psychosocial: This includes feelings, perceptions, beliefs, functional impairment, and role performance.
- Perception: This includes customer perceptions, evaluations, and satisfaction.
- Organization-wide clinical: This includes readmissions, adverse reactions, and deaths.

52. B: The PMHNP should caution the patient to avoid any intake of alcohol because combining the drug with alcohol may result in accumulation of acetaldehyde. Metronidazole inhibits the action of the enzyme aldehyde dehydrogenase, which metabolizes acetaldehyde. This can result in acute alcohol intolerance syndrome.

53. D: Health Status Survey (SF-36 or SF-12) is a tool that provides a client's self-assessment of functional health and quality-of-life issues. Patient Health Questionnaire (PHQ) is used to screen patients and monitor conditions related to mental health disorders, such as depression and anxiety, and substance abuse. Post-Deployment Clinical Assessment Tool (PDCAT) is used to screen returning military for mental health and substance abuse problems related to deployment, including PTSD, depression, anxiety, and alcoholism. The Barthel Index assesses the functional ability of older adults in relation to activities of daily living.

54. D: Pain appears to be driving this patient to suicidal ideation, so the best response is to first directly address the comment to determine the severity of suicidal ideation by asking if the patient has a plan to hurt himself. After the immediate risk assessment, the NP should find ways to alleviate the cause of this patient's distress by offering to work together to find better ways to manage the pain. Many people fear pain more than death, and patients have a right (legal and moral) to be free of pain at the end-of-life. The NP should assess the type, frequency, and duration of pain and current pain management. In some cases, a change to a stronger medication, such as an opioid, or the addition of adjuvant medications may be indicated. Suicidal ideation should be reported to the attending physician and the caregivers should be alerted.

55. A: A data-heavy presentation about progress in performance is most appropriate for administration because administrators are in a position to make decisions and need raw data; however, the presentation should be modified for others. For example, graphs and charts may be used instead of raw data. The PMHNP should assess audience characteristics, including occupation, gender, and education, so that information can be tailored for the audience. For a nonmedical audience, medical jargon should be avoided.

56. B: Unauthorized access: Although EHRs and computerized documentation systems are password protected, providers sometimes share passwords or unwittingly expose their passwords to others when logging in, allowing others to access information about patients. Other forms of data misuse:

- Identity theft: Obtaining identifying information, such as Social Security numbers and credit card numbers, to pose as the other person or access his/her assets.
- Privacy violations: Sharing private information with others, such as family or friends.
- Security breach: Lack of implementation of proper security safeguards and security design, especially when various business associates, such as billing companies, have access to private information, which they misuse.

57. B: Treatment that may be indicated to reduce the breakdown of levodopa is adding entacapone (Comtan), a COMT inhibitor. The COMT enzyme metabolizes levodopa, so a COMT inhibitor slows metabolism to minimize the drug's "wearing off" so that blood levels are maintained until administration of the next dose of levodopa, reducing the on-off phenomenon.

58. D: AIMS detects and evaluates tardive dyskinesia, a common adverse effect associated with neuroleptics. AIMS consists of 12 items that assess orofacial movements, dyskinesia (extremities and trunk), patient awareness and distress, and dental problems. The Trail Making Test (Parts A and B) involves drawing lines to connect sequential numbers, assesses brain function, and indicates increasing dementia. MMSE and the Mini-Cog both assess cognition and involve memory tasks, such as counting backward and remembering words. They are also used to diagnose and evaluate dementia.

59. C: A primary element of a recovery-oriented approach to treatment is recognition that recovery is nonlinear and that multiple episodes of treatment may be required. Treatment should be person-centered, although family, friends, and community agencies should be included in recovery efforts. Treatment does not need to be voluntary in order to be successful. A recovery-oriented approach recognizes that there are multiple approaches to recovery and that a single approach may not serve all individuals.

60. A: In general, medication does little to alleviate inappropriate behavior in patients with dementia, which is best managed by supervision, distracting the patient, or observing for patterns (such as pulling at clothes) that occurs with inappropriate behavior in order to prevent or manage the behavior. Patients with dementia or cognitive impairment may exhibit inappropriate sexual behavior. They may undress, masturbate, request sexual favors, use obscene language, and behave aggressively. The reason for this regression is not clear and behavior may be out of character for the individual but prompted by lack of inhibition and decreased reasoning ability.

61. B: A patient who has been treated for depression with an MAO inhibitor is showing inadequate response and adverse effects, so the PMHNP wants the patient to begin taking an SSRI. The nurse practitioner should stop the MAO inhibitor and wait at least 14 days to start the SSRI. Taking the MAO inhibitor with a medication that increases serotonin levels may cause serotonin syndrome, which may result in fever, chills, anxiety, and confusion.

62. C: The purpose of having a team is so that the work is shared, but leaders can defeat themselves by taking on too much of the workload. Additionally, failure to delegate shows an inherent distrust in team members. Delegation includes:

- Assessing the skills and available time of the team members, determining if a task is suitable for an individual
- Assigning tasks, with clear instructions that include explanation of objectives and expectations, including a timeline
- Ensuring that the tasks are completed properly and on time by monitoring progress but not micromanaging
- Reviewing the final results and recording outcomes

63. D: The first place to begin in developing strategies to improve participation is to survey participants to determine what they feel positive and negative about and eligible patients to determine why they have failed to participate. The survey results can then be used to formulate changes.

64. A: The most likely cause is neuroleptic malignant syndrome, which is a life-threatening complication of neuroleptics. The olanzapine should be discontinued immediately and supportive care provided.

65. C: The best solution is to provide educational programs about research and evidence-based practice (EBP). As staff members become more familiar with research methods and EBP and better able to actively engage in research, they are likely to become more supportive and feel less threatened by changes.

66. B: The primary purpose of the Patient Self-Determination Act is to ensure that patients give informed consent. Patients should be apprised of all options for treatment and all reasonable risks and any complications that might be life-threatening or increase morbidity. The American Medical Association has established the following guidelines for informed consent:

- Explanation of diagnosis
- Nature of, and reason for, treatment or procedure
- Risks and benefits
- Alternative options (regardless of cost or insurance coverage)
- Risks and benefits of alternative options
- Risks and benefits of not having a treatment or procedure
- Providing informed consent is a requirement of all states

67. A: The NP should monitor the child's nutritional status (including height and weight) and sleeping patterns. Methylphenidate depresses appetite, and the child's nutritional intake may be inadequate for a growing child. Additionally, the drug often causes insomnia, so adjusting the dosage or time of administration may be indicated to ensure adequate rest. Suicidal ideation may occur with adolescents.

68. D: This threatens external validity because of subject reactivity (the Hawthorne effect). Behavior often changes when patients recognize that they are being studied.

99

69. A: Steps to conflict resolution include:

- First, allow both sides to present their side of conflict without bias, maintaining a focus on opinions rather than individuals.
- Encourage cooperation through negotiation and compromise.
- Maintain the focus, providing guidance to keep the discussions on track and avoid arguments.
- Evaluate the need for renegotiation, formal resolution process, or third party.

The best time for conflict resolution is when differences emerge but before open conflict and hardening of positions occur. The PMHNP must pay close attention to the people and problems involved, listen carefully, and reassure those involved that their points of view are understood.

70. C: Justice is the ethical principle that relates to the distribution of the limited resources of healthcare benefits to the members of society. These resources must be distributed fairly. This issue may arise if there is only 1 bed left and 2 patients. Justice comes into play in deciding which patient should stay and which should be transported or otherwise cared for. The decision should be made according to what is best or most just for the patients and not colored by personal bias.

71. D: A court order authorizes disclosure of a patient's personal health information. In some cases, this court order may cover only restricted information rather than an entire health record. A subpoena is issued to advise a person that he or she must give testimony in court or in a deposition. A subpoena duces tecum is similar but requires the person to bring specific documents to court. A warrant authorizes an action, such as a search.

72. B: The initial response of the PMHNP should be to order a complete chem-panel, which will include a serum glucose level. Diabetes mellitus is a common cause of impotence in adult men, and the patient also has increased thirst and urinary frequency, which are common symptoms of diabetes.

73. C: The PMHNP's scope of practice is outlined by the state board of nursing and Nurse Practice Act. Advance practice nurses, such as a nurse practitioner or certified nurse specialist, are those who have completed additional education in an accredited nursing program (usually at a master's level) and have received certification with a national certifying organization, such as the American Nurses Credentialing Center. The American Nurses Association and the American Academy of Nurse Practitioners are professional organizations that may help to set standards but do not have legal authority to determine scope of practice.

74. B: While it is common practice to blame the individual responsible for committing an error, in a just culture, the practice is to look at the bigger picture and to try to determine what characteristics of the system are at fault, leading to the error. For example, there may be inadequate staffing, excessive overtime, unclear orders, mislabeling, or other problems that contribute. A just culture differentiates among human error, which results in consoling the person who committed the error; at-risk behavior, which results in coaching to prevent further error; and reckless behavior, which results in punitive action.

75. A: The PMHNP should recognize that these findings may indicate abnormal brain functioning in the parietal lobes. The parietal lobes govern sensory perception as well as the ability to follow directions, tell time, and dress oneself.

76. B: Stage III. Tanner stages for females:

Stages of breast development	Stages of pubic hair
1. Only nipple raised above chest	1. No pubic hair
2. Breast budding	2. Soft, downy hair along labia majora
3. Breast and areola enlarge	3. Sparse dark hair along the labia majora
4. Areola enlarges and may form a secondary elevation	4. Heavy, coarse pubic hair about labia majora
5. Full breasts with pigmented areola and projecting nipples	5. Adult distribution of pubic hair extending laterally and superiorly

77. D: Prior to discharge, the PMHNP should assist the patient to anticipate and cope with pressures. Role playing may be particularly helpful to assist the patient to plan strategies for dealing with offers of drugs or alcohol and alternative methods of handling stressful situations. While avoiding fellow substance abusers or enablers is ideal, it is not always possible.

78. C: If the PMHNP is planning a psychoeducation program for a group of patients with schizophrenia, the most important topic to cover is medication compliance. Patients should have a clear understanding of the purpose of the medications and the risk of noncompliance. Patients who are noncompliant are at increased risk of relapse of symptoms, suicide, and hospitalization. Compliance often is impacted by lack of insight into the disease process, substance abuse, and cognitive impairment.

79. A: Designing a performance improvement plan includes strategic planning for organization-wide participation and collaborative activities, which may be department/discipline specific or interdisciplinary. The plan must be consistent with vision and mission statements and goals and objectives. All performance activities must be referenced to the specific strategic goals or objectives that are part of the mission and vision statements. If there is a disparity, the vision and mission statements may need to be adjusted or the focus of the improvement activities changed.

80. B: According to Erikson's psychosocial theory and stages of development, a 30-year-old man who remains very insecure and dependent on his parents and still lives at home has probably not successfully achieved the stage of identity vs role confusion, which usually occurs during adolescence from age 12-20. The major tasks during this stage are to integrate tasks of earlier stages (developing trust, self-control, sense of purpose, and self-confidence) and to develop a strong sense of the independent self.

81. D: If a 17-year-old patient has been taking fluoxetine for 10 days and feels there is no improvement, the PMHNP should reassure the patient that response often takes 4 weeks. Because the patient is an adolescent, the risk for suicide is increased, so the patient and patient's family should be advised to note any suicidal ideation. Taking fluoxetine in the evening increases the risk of nervousness and insomnia associated with the drug.

82. A: If a patient has agreed to begin treatment with disulfiram, the patient should be aware that drinking alcohol may result in severe illness. Patients must abstain from drinking for 12 hours before initiating treatment. Disulfiram interferes with the breakdown of acetaldehyde from ethanol, so the acetaldehyde level increases, resulting in a syndrome that can include flushing, head and neck pain, severe nausea and vomiting, thirst, excessive perspiration, tachycardia, hyperventilation, weakness, and blurred vision. Some people may develop more severe symptoms, such as myocardial infarction, acute heart failure, and/or respiratory depression.

83. C: A cognitive behavioral therapy (CBT) approach that focuses on relapse prevention for drug use disorders will likely help patients identify situations that make them vulnerable to relapse. Therapy may include training in behavioral skills and the use of cognitive interventions to assist patients in identifying triggers or situations that result in relapse, as well as to provide tools they can use if faced with a situation that is placing them at risk, such as when associates are engaging in addictive behavior.

84. B: When developing a plan of care for a patient with bulimia nervosa, the PMHNP should include instructions that after the patient finishes eating a meal, an attendant should stay with the patient for an hour to prevent the patient from purging. Restoring the patient to normal weight and nutritional status is essential, so the patient must adhere to a diet plan developed by a dietician and be monitored in a structured but supportive environment.

85. A: These signs and symptoms indicate probable somatic symptom disorder. Patients with somatic symptom disorder also often have anxiety disorder. Patients actually perceive pain and feel ill even though no physical cause for symptoms can be identified.

86. D: The initial step in helping the patient quit using through a self-help program should be to help the patient progress beyond the state of Precontemplation with a brief intervention, which may include educating him and helping motivate him to change. Studies have shown that failure rates are high if patients attempt change from a baseline Precontemplation stage (92%) with the failure rate decreasing if the patient begins at Contemplation (85%) or Preparation (75%).

87. C: If a patient's electronic health record indicates that she has a negative variance to the clinical pathway, this means that she has failed to achieve a desired state on the projected timeline. If a negative variance occurs, the PMHNP should carefully assess the patient's plan of care and progress notes to determine what factors contributed to the variance. A positive variance occurs when the patient has responded more quickly than the projected timeline.

88. D: Considering para-verbal communication, if a person speaks rapidly and loudly in a high-pitched voice, the listener is likely to feel that the speaker is angry. If a person speaks slowly and in a low-pitched monotone voice, the listener is likely to feel that the speaker is bored with the conversation. Para-verbal communication refers to the cadence of speech (slow, fast, deliberate) as well as the tone (low-pitched, high-pitched, monotone, trembling voice) and volume (loud, quiet). Para-verbal communication often communicates the feelings of the speaker, even though that may be unintentional.

89. A: If a patient has persistent delusions of persecution, the first step in helping the patient to manage the delusions is to establish a trusting relationship. This is especially important because delusions of persecution may include healthcare providers. It is important to avoid arguing about the patient's beliefs but to state doubt, "I haven't seen the nurse talking about you behind your back," in a matter-of-fact manner. The patient should be encouraged to talk about the delusions before acting on them and to engage in reality testing.

90. B: According to the DSM-5-TR, a patient can be diagnosed with schizophrenic spectrum with only 1 symptom if this symptom is severe delusions or hallucinations, such as hearing ongoing comments or 2 voices. Otherwise, 2 out of the 5 characteristic symptoms (delusions, hallucinations, disorganized speech, disorganized/catatonic behavior/negative symptoms) associated with schizophrenia must be present with at least 1 of the symptoms from the first 3 (delusions, hallucinations, disorganized speech). DSM-5 eliminated subtypes (such as paranoid) of schizophrenia.

91. C: If a patient with generalized anxiety disorder wants to try complementary therapy in addition to medication, the complementary therapy that is most likely to provide some relief of symptoms is relaxation/visualization. However, response is individualized and almost all interventions may have some placebo effect, so some patients report some relief of symptoms with aromatherapy and acupuncture. Yoga is also relaxing and helpful to some patients. There is little evidence to support homeopathy.

92. D: Per SAMHSA guidelines, Suboxone (buprenorphine/naloxone) is administered (at a dose of 2 to 4 mg) in the context of moderate symptoms of opioid withdrawal (represented by a COWS score of >12) with at least 12 hours passing since the last short-acting opioid was taken (24 hours in the context of longer-acting opioids such a heroin). It can then be given every 2 to 4 hours if withdrawal symptoms have not subsided with a maximum daily dose of 8 mg.

93. A: These are indications of bipolar II. Bipolar II must include at least 1 major depressive episode lasting 2 weeks or more and at least 1 episode of hypomania lasting a week or more but does not include episodes of mania or mixed episodes.

94. B: The ethnic group that is most likely to believe that neurobiological disorder is the result of a loss of self-control or punishment for bad behavior is Japanese American. Puerto Ricans often believe that neurobiological disorders result from heredity or from prolonged suffering. Chinese are more likely to believe that neurobiological disorders result from evil spirits or a lack of harmony in emotions. Mexican Americans attribute neurobiological disorders to a variety of causes, including God, spirituality, and interpersonal relationships.

95. C: The patient is probably experiencing denial, an ego defense mechanism. Denial occurs when a patient refuses to acknowledge a painful truth, such as a diagnosis of bipolar disorder. Denial may also include the failure to recognize the behavior or attitudes that allow problems to continue.

96. C: The NP should respect the patient's request. Patients' rights are not determined by who is paying for care but remain with the person. Unless the patient has been declared incompetent in a court proceeding and her parents granted conservatorship, the patient can deny them visitation.

97. A: When choosing a medication to treat a patient with generalized anxiety disorder when rapid onset is desired because of severity of the patient's condition, the best choice is likely clonazepam, which is a long-acting benzodiazepine. Benzodiazepines have rapid onset, usually 1 week or less, so patients may have faster relief of symptoms. Antidepressants, such as venlafaxine and fluoxetine, have a longer period to onset, usually 4 weeks. Onset for buspirone is 2-4 weeks, so it is often given with a benzodiazepine initially.

98. D: The appropriate intervention for a nursing diagnosis of "disturbed thought processes" is to orient the patient to reality frequently and in various ways, such as by placing clocks within view and large signs as reminders. Explanations should be kept simple to avoid overloading the patient, and the PMHNP should speak slowly and in a quiet voice to avoid agitating the patient. The patient should not be encouraged to discuss the delusions but should be encouraged to discuss real events or people.

99. C: The first priority should be to remove the infant from the patient's care because the patient has admitted hating the child and has depersonalized the child by referring to her as "it." Additionally, a patient with severe postpartum depression is at risk for postpartum psychosis, which may further increase risk to the infant.

100. B: While laws may vary slightly from one state to another in relation to involuntary commitment, generally probable cause is present if a person is a threat to self or others (and usually the threat must be imminent). A second criterion is usually that the person is too disabled to provide self-care; however, this last criterion can be interpreted in a wide variety of ways (the reason so many mentally ill individuals are homeless and living on the streets) and is rarely used.

101. D: This patient has signs and symptoms consistent with Wernicke-Korsakoff syndrome, which is associated with alcoholism: confusion, apathy, antegrade and retrograde memory loss, disorientation, disheveled appearance, malnourishment, ataxia with short gait and wide-based stance, nystagmus, and impaired ocular movements. Treatment is with thiamine, usually beginning with parenteral administration for up to a week followed by oral medication. Patients should show improvement within a week but may need long-term care, depending on the severity of the condition.

102. A: This may constitute defamation of character since the information was detrimental to the patient's reputation. Defamation of character generally involves accusations that are malicious or false. Sharing information about the patient is a breach of confidentiality. If the nurse practitioner had put the information in writing, this would represent libel as opposed to slander, which involves orally giving malicious or false information.

103. C: The most effective method of advocating for the value and role of the PMHNP is to conduct clinical research and present findings to multiple groups, such as administration, staff members, patients, and the public. Showing value is more likely to have an effect than talking about it or insisting on it. Conducting research is also a good way to show the value of evidence-based practice and to encourage others to participate in research.

104. D: When working with a patient with conduct disorder, limit setting includes (1) informing the patient of limits, (2) explaining the consequences of noncompliance, and (3) stating expected behaviors. Application of limit setting must be consistent and carried out by all staff members at all times. Consequences must be individualized and must have meaning for the patient so that he is motivated to avoid them. Negotiating a written agreement that can be referred to can prevent conflicts if the patient tries to change the limits.

105. A: An appropriate response by the PMHNP is: "What evidence do you have that you are stupid?" The goal of CBT is to identify cognitive distortions, help the patient to test reality, and correct the distorted beliefs. Patients are taught the skills needed to challenge negative thoughts and replace them with more rational and positive thoughts.

106. A: The effect of the Medicare prospective payment system on health care has been that a primary concern about patient care is discharge and readmission. Organizations are paid not for actual costs but rather a fixed fee based on a particular diagnosis, so early discharge and decreased utilization of services is a financial advantage to an organization, but this must be balanced against the penalty for early readmission if a patient's needs were not met during hospitalization.

107. D: The National Quality Forum's (NQF) Serious Reportable Events (SREs) are those events that are harmful to patients. The SREs are divided into different areas of focus. Those events that focus on Patient Protection are especially applicable to psychiatric-mental health nursing. These events include (1) discharge of a patient unable to make decisions to an unauthorized person, (2) death or serious injury related to elopement/disappearance, and (3) suicide, attempted suicide, or self-harm resulting in serious injury while hospitalized.

108. A: The electrolyte imbalance that the PMHNP should be most concerned about is hypokalemia, which can lead to ventricular arrhythmias and cardiac arrest. Other indications of hypokalemia include lethargy, weakness, nausea and vomiting, muscle cramps, hypotension, and tetany. Normal value for potassium is 3.5-5.5 mEq/L with hypokalemia less than 3.5 mEq/L. Critical value is less than 2.5 mEq/L.

109. B: The type of grief response that the patient is exhibiting is conflicted grief, one form of complicated grief. This type of grief is most common if the relationship between the deceased and the patient involved conflict.

110. C: If a 26-year-old female patient with a history of anorexia nervosa has an ideal body weight of 130 pounds, the weight at which the patient will first be diagnosed with a relapse is 107 pounds, which is 82% of ideal (less than 85% is diagnostic). Patients with a history of anorexia nervosa often retain some body image concerns and should be routinely monitored to ensure they are maintaining an adequate body weight.

111. A: The patient must have weekly white blood cell counts for at least 6 months, then every 2 weeks for an additional 6 months, and then every month thereafter. Clozapine can cause agranulocytosis, and the patient may not be able to take the drug if his absolute neutrophil count drops. Clozapine has multiple adverse effects, so the patient must be monitored carefully.

112. D: Families should be assisted to develop a crisis safety plan that includes recognizing the signs of an impending crisis and using de-escalation techniques to defuse the situation. De-escalation techniques include avoiding touching the patient without permission and quietly describing any action before carrying it out so as not to further alarm the patient. The family member should remain calm, speak quietly, listen, express concern, avoid arguing and making continuous eye contact, keep environmental stimulation low, allow the person adequate space, and offer suggestions but avoid taking control.

113. C: A patient who complains that the doctor implanted a controlling microchip in his arm and that he needs to cut it out is experiencing a delusion of control because he believes that his behavior is under the control of someone or something else. With delusions of persecution, the patient feels threatened or frightened and believes someone or something wants to harm him. With a somatic delusion, the patient has unrealistic ideas about his/her body while, with a nihilistic delusion, the patient believes that an important aspect of reality (the self, the world) no longer exists.

114. B: The type of aphasia that is most common to frontotemporal dementia is primary progressive aphasia (PPA). PPA results from a neurodegenerative process, which also occurs with Alzheimer disease. There are subtypes of PPA, so the clinical picture may vary somewhat, but patients usually exhibit halting speech, decreased language use, difficulty finding words, mixing up the order of words, mispronouncing words, and substituting words. Patients have difficulty understanding and using language, writing, and reading with progressive and irreversible deterioration.

115. A: When developing an education plan for a group of homeless patients with alcohol use disorder, the most important information to include is probably information about community resources, including shelters, food banks, free meals, free clinics, and self-help groups, such as Alcoholics Anonymous. Inpatient care is often an unrealistic goal for homeless people with few or no financial resources unless care is mandated by the courts and covered by government programs. Patients who are homeless and addicted often have multiple problems, including dual diagnoses, which make personal responsibility difficult to achieve.

116. D: The most common reason for nonadherence to medical treatment for neurobiological disorders is that the patient believes he or she does not have a neurobiological disorder and can manage without medication. Many patients also are dependent on alcohol or drugs and may be advised to avoid alcohol or drugs with medications, so they stop the medications. Adverse effects of medications can be troubling and may cause some patients to stop taking them. Patients may stop treatment if they are confused, but confusion may also result from decreasing or stopping medication.

117. B: If the PMHNP has suggested a change in procedure based on evidence-based research but has encountered considerable staff resistance, the best approach is to suggest a limited trial period to evaluate the effect of the change. Resistance to change is very common, so it is important to try to gain acceptance rather than to point fingers or use coercion as the first strategy. A trial period is often less threatening and provides an opportunity to gather data to support the change.

118. C: The most common comorbid condition associated with schizophrenia is substance use disorder, sometimes as the result of trying to self-medicate. Patients with schizophrenia also often smoke, so treatment protocols should include drug, alcohol, and smoking cessation. Drug and alcohol use is frequently a factor in nonadherence to treatment plans, especially if it is advised that alcohol or drugs should be avoided with medications. Patients with schizophrenia may also have the comorbidities of post-traumatic stress disorder, panic disorder, and obsessive-compulsive disorder, complicating treatment approaches.

119. D: According to the Centers for Disease Control and Prevention (CDC), patients who inject drugs should receive immunizations for hepatitis A and B, which are transmitted through sharing of needles contaminated with blood. There is no vaccine available for hepatitis C although patients should be screened for hepatitis C because they are at risk for the disease. There is also not any immunization for HIV/AIDS, although patients may also need screening for HIV. Immunization for herpes zoster is not associated with injection drug use.

120. A: Patients with Tourette's syndrome should be assessed for the common comorbidities of attention-deficit/hyperactivity disorder (ADHD) and obsessive-compulsive disorder (OCD) as up to 95% of those with Tourette syndrome have another psychiatric disorder. Medications often used for treatment of ADHD may worsen tic behavior (although this conclusion is controversial) but treating OCD often reduces tics. When determining treatment options, the initial focus is usually on the condition that is causing the most impairment rather than treating more than 1 condition.

121. B: If during an interview the patient blames his boss for his problems and states that the boss is "going to pay," this is an implied threat. Because of the duty to warn those who might be in danger from a patient with mental health issues, the PMHNP should ask directly, "What thoughts have you had about hurting your boss?" in order to assess whether there is a risk of violence.

122. A: The most likely cause of the CNS depression is the combination of a CYP3A4 substrate (alprazolam) with an inhibitor (isoniazid). The inhibitor allows the blood level of the drug to increase to toxic levels because it slows the metabolism of the drug. Symptoms of toxicity usually occur within about a week.

123. C: The PMHNP's first priority should be to protect self and others. Unless the nurse practitioner has had special training in dealing with patients with weapons, he should not attempt to disarm or subdue the patient and should keep something between himself and the patient, such as a pillow or chair, and maintain a distance beyond 4 feet. The PMHNP should summon help and try to clear the room if other patients are present.

124. B: The best approach is to say, "I know you are afraid, but you are safe here." The PMHNP should acknowledge the patient's fears while trying to use grounding techniques to remind the patient that he is safe. The PMHNP should not attempt to reach out to the patient or touch the patient without first asking for permission as this may trigger a violent response.

125. D: Because the toddler's behavior suggests autism spectrum disorder, the initial screening test the PMHNP should recommend is the M-CHAT-R (Modified Checklist for Autism in Toddlers-Revised) for children 16-30 months. This test is available for free and easily self-administered by a caregiver in a few minutes and consists of 20 questions about the child's behavior. Score of 0-2 is low risk; 3-7 is medium risk; and 8-20 is high risk.

126. B: The best response is that this can result in alcohol poisoning. Alcohol breaks down into acetaldehyde, but many Asians lack the enzyme needed to rid the body of acetaldehyde, so it accumulates and causes a severe flushing response. H2 blockers slow the metabolism of alcohol to acetaldehyde but can result in excessive drinking and toxicity because the effects of drinking are delayed.

127. A: Considering Maslow's hierarchy, the order in which the nursing diagnoses for a patient should be prioritized (first to last) is:

1. Physiological needs: deficient fluid volume.
2. Safety needs: Risk for self-injury.
3. Love/belonging needs: sexual dysfunction.
4. Esteem needs: low self-esteem.

Physiological needs, especially those that are critical to life, should always be a top priority. However, prioritizing does not necessarily mean that the first priority must be dealt with before the PMHNP can deal with the second priority because, in reality, many diagnoses may be attended to simultaneously.

128. A: The primary risk factor for alcohol abuse and dependence is genetic predisposition, which comprises about 50% of risk, although other factors may increase or decrease the genetic effects. Substance abuse and dependence clearly run in families, but peer influence and socioeconomic status are also factors. Ethnicity also has an effect with some Native Americans and Asians, especially, lacking enzymes needed to metabolize alcohol.

129. C: In milieu therapy, if a person exhibits inappropriate behavior, the correct response is to help the patient examine the effect the behavior has on others and to discuss more appropriate ways of behaving. With milieu therapy, expectations are that all patients can grow and that all interactions have the potential to be therapeutic. Patients "own" their environment and behavior and must be responsible for both. Peer pressure is used to provide direct feedback, and consequences (punishment/restrictions) are to be avoided.

130. B: The NP must recognize that the most subjective type of review is narrative, which often omits details about research methods and designs. Narrative reviews may be useful for screening to determine what studies to review in more depth but should not be used as evidence because the interpretation may be biased.

131. B: These lab results suggest that the patient's depression may result from hypothyroidism related to thyroid dysfunction. Typically, the TSH level rises to stimulate the thyroid to produce T4, so the levels may remain normal for a while because of the increased TSH or may begin to fall. If thyroid dysfunction was related to pituitary dysfunction, the TSH level would generally be decreased instead of elevated.

132. D: Patients taking lithium for bipolar disease are likely to begin to exhibit signs of toxicity if levels exceed 1.5 mEq/L. Lithium levels should remain between 0.6 and 1.4 mEq/L for adults, a narrow therapeutic range. Levels should be measured about 8-12 hours after the last dose because the half-life ranges from 18-24 hours. Sodium levels should also be monitored and maintained in normal range (135-145 mEq/L).

133. C: When conducting research using a database search for evidence-based practice, the PMHNP should avoid stopwords (*a, an, and, for in, of, the, this*, and *to*). Some databases will indicate a failed search if stopwords are included in a search. Nesting is used to group terms together with parentheses. Wildcards are symbols, such as the ? used in place of 1 or more letters. Truncation is searching with a root instead of entire words, usually followed by a symbol, such as *nurs**.

134. D: If the PMHNP notes a flattening of the patient's nasolabial fold and drooping of the lower eyelids, these findings suggest damage to the 7th cranial (facial) nerve. The 7th cranial nerve should be examined at rest and while the patient is talking to note facial asymmetry or other abnormalities. Examination includes asking the patient to raise the eyebrows, frown, close the eyes tightly, bare upper and lower teeth, smile, and close the mouth and puff out the cheeks.

135. A: While all of these questions may have value, if a person states repeatedly that he wants to die, the most critical question is, "Do you have access to dangerous weapons?" Many patients will acknowledge that they have access to guns or knives, and studies indicate that those with familiarity with weapons, such as members of the military or hunters, have increased risk of carrying through with suicide. It is important to enlist the help of family or friends to secure potential weapons if possible.

136. B: The first essential element in providing trauma-informed care is to recognize the prevalence of trauma and its effects on mental and physical health as well as family and social relationships. Trauma can affect all facets of a patient's life. Over 60% of men and 50% of women have reported trauma, the definition of which may vary widely. What is traumatic to one individual may have little effect on another, but trauma should be viewed within the context of the patient's experience and environment.

137. D: Behaviors that indicate the child is at risk of progress to antisocial personality disorder (APD) include cruelty to animals. While substance abuse is common, it is not necessarily a risk factor for development of APD. For an APD diagnosis, the signs/symptoms must have been present before age 15 and the patient must be at least 18 at time of diagnosis. Other risk factors include stealing, mugging, bullying, starting fires, carrying out sexual assaults, lying habitually, and using weapons against others.

138. C: The Denver Developmental Screening Test II, appropriate for children from birth up to 6 years old, does not test for cognitive ability. The 4 domains covered by the DDST II include language, gross motor skills, personal-social, and fine motor-adaptive skills. DDST II requires about 30 minutes to complete and requires observation of the child and input from parents or caregivers. Both English and Spanish versions are available; however, administering the assessment in a hospital environment in which the child is stressed may interfere with the results.

139. B: The most appropriate action for the nurse practitioner is to carry out a cost-benefit analysis in advance of making the proposal. The purpose of this analysis is to show how costs may be offset by more efficiency, which may increase income.

140. C: The PMHNP should not interrupt a child at play with a direct question, which interferes with the child's process of working out feelings of anxiety and may cause increased stress. A better approach is to use a reflective statement, such as "I see that the little boy in your picture is crying" or "I wonder why the little boy is crying," and leave it to the child to respond or not. Focusing on the picture rather than the child may be less threatening and help him to express feelings and explain why the child in the picture is crying.

141. A: If the PMHNP is observing an interdisciplinary team to determine what works and what does not work, a negative practice is interrupting speakers and interpreting their comments. Team members should also avoid interpreting others' remarks, reacting to feelings rather than facts, jumping to conclusions, and giving unsolicited advice. Open communication and respect for each other are critical elements to positive interactions.

142. C: If the PMHNP plans to access the healthcare system's data warehouse for research purposes, this is referred to as data mining. For data mining, software is used to sort through data and identify patterns or relationships. Data warehouses are very large databases, usually holding all of an organization or system's data. A data mart, by contrast, contains data on a specific topic or for a specific department.

143. D: According to Gestalt therapy (Perls), introjection is the term for a boundary disturbance that involves accepting the beliefs/opinions of other people without questioning them. Retroflection involves turning something/emotions meant for another person or thing back onto the self, often as a protective mechanism. Deflection is a method of interfering with contact or communication. Projection involves attributing impulses/actions to others rather than to themselves and fantasizing about what others may be experiencing.

144. B: This type of alternative dispute resolution is mediation. Mandatory use of mediation or arbitration is often included in employment contracts. Arbitration is a more formal procedure, typically involving presentation of evidence and statements by witnesses, and the resulting decision is usually binding.

145. C: This is a situation in which the ethical principle of autonomy is in conflict with the principle of beneficence. With beneficence, the aim is to do good and serve the needs of the patient by providing a sitter to prevent injury. In this case, this takes precedence over the patient's right to autonomy.

146. D: The response by the PMHNP that exemplifies reflection is: "It sounds as though you have been disappointed many times." Reflection is used to help people to better understand their feelings and emotions about events and may be a statement or a simple question.

147. A: The first step in successfully communicating within and across an organization in order to promote change is to identify key concerns of different individuals and departments and then to address those concerns as part of the initial communication. For example, if a key concern of change is increase in workload, the PMHNP may begin communication by stressing that one goal is to reduce workload. Individuals and, by extension, departments are likely to be more receptive if they perceive benefit.

148. D: If utilizing the FOCUS (find, organize, clarify, uncover, start) model of performance improvement, the initial step is to find what isn't working well in the organization. Organize involves identifying those who understand the problems and forming a performance improvement team. Clarify is to brainstorm and identify methods of solving problems. Uncover is to identify the underlying reasons for problems through analysis, and start is to determine where and how to begin the change process.

149. B: When determining sample size for evidence-based inquiry, according to the "Rule of 10," at least 10 subjects are needed for each variable studied. In this case, there are 4 variables, so 40 subjects are needed. Another method is to apply the "Rule of 30," which means that a subject population should comprise at least 30. A third method of determining sample size is power analysis, which is based on significance level (usually $P = 0.05$) and effect size (estimate of the difference between groups).

150. C: In keeping with professional standards, if the PMHNP wants be become a political activist, an appropriate form of activism would be to write letters/emails to politicians regarding concerns. The nurse practitioner should avoid discussing political matters with patients and should also avoid any perception of coercion, such as through questioning workplace associates or posting political posters in the workplace. The nurse practitioner may choose to become involved in national organizations to promote a political agenda.

151. A: This type of organizational structure is referred to as service-line because all services to mental health patients are under management of one individual. While this structure speeds up decision making and helps clarify purpose, it can result in duplication of services and isolation from other professionals.

152. D: The most appropriate response is, "I can't keep information regarding your health or wellbeing from other team members." This establishes clear parameters, which still allows the patient to discuss some private matters if the patient chooses to do so.

153. D: The best approach is to talk to the child about the traumatic event, allowing the child to express feelings. If the child cannot talk about the event, sometimes the child may express feelings through art, such as drawing pictures, but avoiding the issue is not a good solution.

154. C: The first thing the nurse practitioner should do in preparation for leadership is to study the team members' job descriptions and learn their roles and responsibilities. While roles vary, all members are equally important to a team, and relationships should be based on mutual trust and respect.

155. A: This type of prevention effort is primary. The purpose of primary prevention is to prevent the health problem (in this case addiction) from occurring. Secondary prevention aims to identify substance abuse early and to provide intervention, and tertiary prevention aims to reduce existing conditions and prevent further deterioration.

156. D: A patient with borderline personality disorder is most likely to benefit from dialectical behavioral therapy (DBT), which tries to help the patient replace thinking that views the world as black or white with rational (dialectical) thinking. DBT comprises individual therapy to help the patient develop behavioral goals and to begin self-monitoring, group skills training (core mindfulness skills [mediation], interpersonal skills, emotion modulation skills, and distress tolerance skills), and telephone consultation and support.

157. B: Begin with assessment. When conducting gap analysis, the following steps are followed:

- Assess the current situations/processes and list all important factors
- Identify current outcomes of these situations/processes
- Identify target outcomes

- Outline the processes to be put in place to achieve target outcomes
- Identify the gaps that exist between the present process and the target outcomes
- Identify the resources required to achieve the target outcomes and close the gap

Gap analysis identifies the steps required to move from the current state to a projected state.

158. C: If the PMHNP is conducting a psychiatric exam, homicidal, suicidal, and violence ideations are evaluated as part of examination of the element of abnormal/psychotic thoughts. This element also includes determining whether the patient has delusions, hallucinations, and/or obsessions. Judgment and insight include the ability to identify and understand problems in social activities. Thought processes include the ability to think logically, carry out computations, and use abstract reasoning. Mood and affect include evidence of indications such as depression, mania, hypomania, and labile emotions.

159. A: Most children are potty trained between ages 2 and 3 but some resist training, especially with bowel movements. The best suggestion is to use incentives or disincentives to encourage the child to cooperate, but it is important to avoid simple rewards (candy, toys) or punishments as these may precipitate a battle for control. Incentives that involve actions or experiences, such as being able to watch a movie or to go to a park, are good choices.

160. C: When trying to help patients reduce risk factors, such as drinking and smoking, for which there is little immediate reward (indeed, immediate results may be withdrawal and cravings), the PMHNP should assist the patient to establish short-term and long-term goals. Patients who are working toward a clearly defined goal have purpose and are more likely to stay with a program. It is important that goals be realistic and attainable.

161. D: If taking advantage of neuroplasticity following a traumatic brain injury (TBI), the patient should do repetitive physical exercises/activities. This repetition encourages the development of new pathways in the brain. Neuroplasticity helps to heal the brain in 4 ways:

- Functional map extension: healthy cells surrounding a damaged area take over the function of the missing cells.
- Compensatory masquerade: existing neural pathways reorganize to compensate for damaged ones.
- Homologous region adoption: a new area of the brain takes over the function of a distant damaged area.
- Cross-model reassignment: one sensory area is enhanced to compensate for losses of another sensory area.

162. B: Instrumental relativist orientation. Kohlberg's stages of moral development include:

- Level I (ages 4-10): Punishment and obedience orientation (child recognizes adults as rule givers and that punishment occurs with bad behavior). Instrumental relativist orientation (child may make moral judgments based on what she gets from the decision).
- Level II (ages 10 through adolescence): Interpersonal concordance (child gains approval by helping others). Law and order orientation (child makes moral decisions out of respect for authority or sense of duty).
- Level III (adulthood): Social contract legalist orientation and universal ethical-principle orientation (e.g., justice, equality).

163. A: If the PMHNP wants to effect health policy, the nurse practitioner should begin by gaining information about the system (local, state, federal). For example, the nurse practitioner needs to know which branch of government makes the policy of interest and who is responsible as well as the type of input and research used. Then, a review of the issue, the key stakeholders, and the processes involved should be carried out.

164. C: An organizational structure in which professional and nonprofessional staff members are divided according to the type of work that they do (nursing, laboratory, housekeeping) and staff report to discipline specific managers is classified as functional. This type of organizational structure tends to limit interactions across different disciplines but is often cost-effective. This is one of the most traditional structures, but coordinating activities with different disciplines can be challenging because of different goals and status in the hierarchy.

165. D: If the PMHNP is testing the reliability of 2 staff members' scoring by having them measure the same event together and then comparing their scores, this method tests for equivalence. Testing for interrater reliability is especially important if a number of different individuals are involved in gathering data through observation because otherwise the data may be skewed. Instruments and research methods should be also tested for stability, internal consistency, and external consistency.

166. B: With a consultative style of leadership, the leader presents a decision and welcomes staff members to give input and to pose questions, although the leader rarely changes the decision. With participative leadership, the leader presents a potential decision and makes the final decision based on input. With autocratic leadership, the leader makes and imposes decisions. With democratic leadership, the leader poses a problem and asks staff to come up with a solution.

167. B: When assigning roles to team leaders, the informatics nurse should first consider their education and skills in order to match members to the most appropriate roles because members are more likely to be effective if they are dealing with roles with which they have some familiarity. The members' available time investment is also important to ensure that the members actually have the time needed to carry out the roles. Commitment to team efforts is also important but can be modified by effective or ineffective leadership. Personality types vary widely but should not be a deciding factor.

168. A: Shared governance implies shared decision making, but this can be realized in different ways. A common form of shared governance is for the administration to allow autonomous decision making by specific departments, teams, or groups within an organization regarding issues that apply to them or are within their area of expertise. For example, a unit team may have the authority to establish work schedules for that unit only, and members of a professional development team may be able to make decisions regarding professional development activities. In some cases, shared governance committees communicate with administration and can affect decision making but do not make the final decision.

169. D: This is probably an indication of poor communication. Staff should be apprised of patients' conditions and plans, including those for discharge, and should have input into patient readiness for discharge. The nurse practitioner should ensure that regular communication across disciplines occurs regarding patients at scheduled times, such as through daily rounds.

170. C: If the PMHNP is assigned as care manager for a group of patients, the first task the nurse practitioner should complete is a needs assessment. The nurse practitioner may conduct interviews (patient, family, staff), use questionnaires, and review patient records. In order to manage a patient's care, the nurse practitioner must have a clear idea of the patients' physical and mental health, social circumstances, and support systems.

171. A: An example of passive resistance is agreeing but failing to act, a common method of resistance because the individual does not need to take a public stance against the change. Other passive methods include avoiding any discussion of the change and essentially ignoring it. Active resistance includes organizing resistance, verbally attacking the change, and refusing to make the change.

172. B: In a psychiatric unit, patients are primarily able to exercise power through praise and complaints because these may bring about change. For example, if a patient files a complaint about a staff member, this may bring about disciplinary action. Likewise, if a patient praises a certain intervention, this may help to influence further use of the intervention. Threats and intimidation as well as cooperation and lack of cooperation may bring about a response, but they are not exercises in real power. Rewards and punishments are not generally within the purview of patients.

173. D: The supervisor is likely to note that the nurse practitioner needs improvement in time management so that tasks can be completed during working hours. Staff members are paid for a certain number of hours and it can reflect badly on the administration if members must stay overtime, and unpaid overtime poses ethical problems.

174. C: If 2 nursing positions have been lost, the best solution for assigning patients is to switch to an acuity-based model so that nurses have unequal numbers of patients but essentially equal workloads. A method for assigning acuity level must be developed with input from staff members. Cost cutting is a reality in today's health care, so demanding additional hiring is unlikely to be effective unless cost-effectiveness can be demonstrated.

175. B: If the PMHNP notes that team members seem to have difficulty with time management, the best method of dealing with this is to begin with a time log for a week. People often underestimate or overestimate the time needed for tasks, so a time log presents concrete evidence of actual time spent in productive and nonproductive activities and can help to determine where changes can benefit staff members.

Tell Us Your Story

We at Mometrix would like to extend our heartfelt thanks to you for letting us be a part of your journey. It is an honor to serve people from all walks of life, people like you, who are committed to building the best future they can for themselves.

We know that each person's situation is unique. But we also know that, whether you are a young student or a mother of four, you care about working to make your own life and the lives of those around you better.

That's why we want to hear your story.

We want to know why you're taking this test. We want to know about the trials you've gone through to get here. And we want to know about the successes you've experienced after taking and passing your test.

In addition to your story, which can be an inspiration both to us and to others, we value your feedback. We want to know both what you loved about our book and what you think we can improve on.

The team at Mometrix would be absolutely thrilled to hear from you! So please, send us an email at tellusyourstory@mometrix.com or visit us at mometrix.com/tellusyourstory.php and let's stay in touch.